ADVANCE PRAISE FOR
PCOS IS MY POWER

"I am absolutely elated to see Cory Ruth turn her PCOS journey and educational skills into a relatable format that a best friend would give on a Saturday night over wine, a bonfire, and a pile of recipes and research articles. **This book will forever change the entrance into womanhood with PCOS from one of shame and fear into one of hope and empowerment.** By harnessing a true understanding of actionable ways to take charge of PCOS, women can work to restore their reproductive health, light-years beyond what is offered with the current standard of care."

—**NAOMI WHITTAKER**, MD

"As a holistic gynecologist, I find PCOS to be one of the most difficult problems to treat. Cory Ruth is a leader in the field of PCOS, and with *PCOS Is My Power*, we finally have **a comprehensive, medically backed approach to PCOS** that will revolutionize how we combat this difficult yet common women's health issue. I will recommend it to all my PCOS patients."

—**SHAWN TASSONE**, MD, PhD, and author of *The Hormone Balance Bible*

"As someone who's learned to support my PCOS symptoms with food, *PCOS Is My Power* felt like **a breath of fresh air.** Cory Ruth doesn't just explain the science—she also serves up real, nourishing solutions that taste as good as they feel. Her recipes are **approachable and empowering,** and her insights into how food can truly reset our hormones are exactly what our community has been waiting for."

—**CAILEE FISCHER**, creator of @CaileeEats

"Cory Ruth is **a beacon of hope for women with PCOS.** While most healthcare providers only focus on medical treatments for PCOS, Cory offers hundreds of lifestyle tips and tricks to those seeking a holistic approach. This book helps you understand not just what PCOS is, but how to address many drivers of its symptoms, leading to long-term, lasting PCOS management. Filled with supplement ideas and recipe inspo, *PCOS Is My Power* is sure to become a staple on the shelves of PCOS sufferers and PCOS health providers."

—**HANNAH MUEHL**, MS, RDN, PA-C

PCOS IS MY POWER

Your Guide to Understanding PCOS,
Fixing Your Hormones,
and Resetting Your Health

CORY RUTH

Foreword by Dr. Jolene Brighten

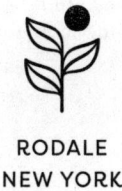

RODALE
NEW YORK

Rodale Books
An imprint of Random House
A division of Penguin Random House LLC
1745 Broadway, New York, NY 10019
rodalebooks.com | randomhousebooks.com
penguinrandomhouse.com

A Rodale Trade Paperback Original

Copyright © 2026 by Cory Ruth

Penguin Random House values and supports copyright. Copyright fuels creativity, encourages diverse voices, promotes free speech, and creates a vibrant culture. Thank you for buying an authorized edition of this book and for complying with copyright laws by not reproducing, scanning, or distributing any part of it in any form without permission. You are supporting writers and allowing Penguin Random House to continue to publish books for every reader. Please note that no part of this book may be used or reproduced in any manner for the purpose of training artificial intelligence technologies or systems.

Rodale & Plant with colophon is a registered trademark of Penguin Random House LLC.

Names: Ruth, Cory author | Brighten, Jolene writer of foreword
Title: PCOS is my power / by Cory Ruth, RDN; foreword by Dr. Jolene Brighten.
Other titles: Polycystic Ovary Syndrome is my power
Description: New York, NY : Rodale, [2026] | Includes bibliographical references and index. |
Identifiers: LCCN 2025035843 (print) | LCCN 2025035844 (ebook) | ISBN 9780593980668 trade paperback |
ISBN 9780593980675 Ebook
Subjects: LCSH: Ruth, Cory—Psychology | Polycystic ovary syndrome—Treatment--Popular works |
Polycystic ovary syndrome—Psychological aspects—Popular works
Classification: LCC RG480.S7 R88 2026 (print) | LCC RG480.S7 (ebook)

Printed in the United States of America on acid-free paper

1st Printing

BOOK TEAM: Production editor: Cassie Gitkin • Managing editor: Allison Fox •
Production manager: Chanler Harris • Copy editor: Hope Clarke •
Proofreaders: Liz Carbonell, Cyrus Chin, Marisa Crumb, Leda Scheintaub

Book design by Ralph Fowler

FIRST PAPERBACK EDITION

The authorized representative in the EU for product safety and compliance
is Penguin Random House Ireland, Morrison Chambers, 32 Nassau Street,
Dublin D02 YH68, Ireland. https://eu-contact.penguin.ie

To my truly wonderful husband, for always
rallying behind my half-crazy ideas and never
protesting a lasagna made with zucchini ribbons.

To my three incredible children, who bring me purpose,
joy, laughter, and some premature gray hairs.

To my parents, who inspire me to chase my dreams
and continue to empower and educate other
women with my same diagnosis.

CONTENTS

A rapid increase in weight at puberty that you have struggled with most of your life, a dodgy period that you counted yourself lucky you didn't have to deal with often, or cystic acne that you were told was just your hormones may have been part of your coming-of-age story. Maybe your experience was going on the Pill to "fix all the hormone issues," only to discover years later, when you struggled to get pregnant, that there was more to the acne and irregular periods than your doctor may have said. Or maybe you're that one-in-ten of polycystic ovary syndrome (PCOS) patients who managed a diagnosis but hasn't been satisfied with the treatment results or lack thereof.

The truth is, healing symptoms of PCOS doesn't look the same for every person. This is why the single-drug or one-size-fits-all approach is not only ineffective but in some cases harmful. Those with PCOS are at a three- to sixfold increased risk of developing an eating disorder, in part due to advice received from well-meaning medical providers, personal trainers, or self-proclaimed health gurus. Women with PCOS don't need another fad diet—they need evidence-based nutrition strategies that look to support overall health rather than a "weight loss at any cost" agenda.

In my clinical experience, the most effective management of PCOS is patient-centered and integrates the best of lifestyle therapies, nutrition interventions, and medications, if needed. In fact, the 2023 International Evidence-based Guidelines for the Assessment and Management of PCOS state that a healthy lifestyle that includes nutrition and exercise interventions should be recommended to all women with PCOS. But despite these recommendations, few women with PCOS receive that level of support.

A multifaceted disease impacting every system of the body, PCOS remains one of the most misunderstood conditions in women's medicine, and because of that, many women struggle to find a practitioner they can partner with. For all these reasons, there is a need for a book of this caliber within the PCOS community.

What Cory Ruth has created within this book is a beacon of hope for those navigating the complexities of this condition. She draws upon her expertise and experience to provide you with a clear understanding of PCOS, debunking myths and misconceptions along the way. From the science behind PCOS to strategies for symptom management and lifestyle interventions, this book offers a comprehensive road map to help you effectively address the symptoms of PCOS.

As you embark on this journey, I encourage you to approach it through the lens of what is true for you. Whether you are newly diagnosed with PCOS or have been living with it for years, know that you are not alone. Use the stories of real women who have reversed their PCOS symptoms to inspire and encourage you on your journey. Each story is a reminder that PCOS does present challenges, but with the right strategies specific to your needs, you can overcome them.

May this book serve as a guiding light for you as you seek understanding, support, and empowerment in your journey with PCOS.

Dr. Jolene Brighten, NMD, FABNE,
Certified Sexuality Counselor

PCOS
IS MY POWER

INTRODUCTION

Has anyone ever looked forward to getting her period?

Well, I'll tell you a secret.

I do. Only because, for FOREVER, it was an elusive, sneaky b*tch that never wanted to come on time. When it did arrive, it never seemed to *leave*. My period was like the long-term hookup who couldn't decide if he wanted to commit or swipe on Tinder for eternity. Let me take you back to the start of my relationship with my on-again, off-again hot mess of a cycle.

Long ago, in a faraway land called Sacramento, California, I was a high school sophomore in the locker room with my friends. After we changed from sweaty gym clothes, my bestie leaned over and whispered, "I'm gonna get my period this Saturday! Looks like I'll be eating ice cream in sweats this weekend."

I looked at her like she was an alien with information zapped to her from the future. *How did she know that? What magic allowed her to know her period was coming ON SATURDAY?*

I was stunned. My Auntie Flo had been dead set on random for the past three years. Even though I had started getting my period at thirteen, and *everyone* told me it was supposed to be initially wonky, mine never evened out. EVER. That twenty-eight-day cycle they taught in sex ed? Bah! That seemed just as ridiculous as a teacher telling me the tooth fairy was real.

Even then I knew something was off. In my head, a voice said things like *Something is seriously wrong with you. Something is wrong with your body. You aren't normal.*

This shame spiral continued for a few years as everyone else matured into late puberty, while my body never managed to get a stupid period right. If I needed *any more* evidence for my freakishness, all I had to do was look at my sheets at home: stained with random, uncontrollable spotting. For weeks, I would bleed through super tampons and pads, and then Aunt Flo would disappear, only to pop up again on the afternoon of the pool party I had been dying to attend.

Every random period proved I was just . . . broken. My body, it seemed, was destined to get a D in functioning, and as a student who loved straight-A marks, I felt like a freak and a failure.

And I know you've felt that way, too.

WHAT I WISH I KNEW

If only I could go back and hug that little teenager now. I would tell her that it took me another decade to figure out that *nothing* was wrong with me.

I would scoop her up and explain we had polycystic ovary syndrome (PCOS). I would calmly say that PCOS is one of the world's most common female hormonal disorders—nearly one in every ten women has it. I wasn't a freak, a failure, or even at fault for having this disorder. No, I just had something a lot of other women had that *nobody talks enough about.*

Then, I would tell my younger self that it would take me years of personal and professional research to understand: PCOS IS NOT A DEATH SENTENCE. It's a treatable condition that can be managed through lifestyle and dietary changes. Practices like getting a regular movement routine; eating plenty of protein, fat, and fiber; and managing one's blood sugar can seriously move the needle on unwanted symptoms—like the period from hell.

Finally, I would tell her even though PCOS is the leading cause of infertility worldwide and is one of the most gaslit female medical conditions, getting a diagnosis wasn't the end of my life. Despite it, I would grow up to ovulate on a regular cycle, have beautiful babies, and not let this condition define me. No matter what mood swings came my way, my PCOS would not dictate my relationship with my happiness. Instead, it would be the air under my wings that made me fly. And babes, it can be the same for you.

WHO AM I?

My name is Cory Ruth, and I am a PCOS dietitian and weight loss and fertility specialist. I went from being a confused kid in a locker room struggling with weight gain, hair loss, and anxiety to a woman who took full charge of her health. Not only that, I graduated at the top of my class in my master's of nutrition program. In 2018, I founded my viral practice, The Women's Dietitian, which is dedicated to helping women with PCOS thrive. Through carefully curated research, I have helped thousands of women with PCOS regulate their periods, lose all the weight they wanted, have healthy, beautiful babies, heal their hormones, and live balanced lives (including eating ooey-gooey burgers!) even *with* a PCOS diagnosis. With grit and creativity, I have become one of the leading authorities in the PCOS nutrition space, and I help women achieve remarkable results with their health.

The secret weapon? Knowledge.

I know my patients' pain because I have PCOS, too, and I've been where they've been on their health journey—but I've come out the other side. With my guidance, my patients have made profound shifts in their life through simple and sustainable lifestyle changes: a balanced diet, an intentional supplement regimen, exercise, and stress management. Each of these changes is achievable and affordable.

Despite the fact that women with PCOS are at a three times higher risk for anxiety and depression than those without the diagnosis, AND more than half of women with PCOS develop type 2 diabetes by age forty, AND 80 percent of PCOS warriors struggle with obesity, my patients have leveled out their blood sugar, lost hundreds of pounds collectively, gained mastery over their flare-ups, started ovulating on regular cycles, and had sweet little babies without IVF.

I'm so proud not only of their changes but of their shift in perspective and lifestyle, which has allowed them to achieve lasting results.

THE CASE STUDIES

In this book, we will explore five stories of bad*ss patients whom I have helped. We will dive into where they were in their diagnosis journey *before* working with me, how their symptoms improved based on the guidelines I offered, and what myths we had to B-U-S-T to get them to their healthiest selves.

Through these narratives, I aim to explore how anyone can walk through the darkest parts of their PCOS, reboot their health, and become who they want to be.

I'm not saying it's easy, but it's possible. And you can do it, too.

BUT IT'S NOT FAIR!

Baby girl, I *know* having PCOS can be a real bummer. Personally, my PCOS was the common variable behind some of the lowest moments of my life. I gained nearly fifty pounds during college with the help of beer, burritos, and trying *one million* different birth control methods that ruined my libido, made my weight skyrocket, and left me feeling depressed and hopeless.

Then, after finally getting a diagnosis, I cried uncontrollably in a bathroom when my doctor offhandedly told me I would need "significant medical intervention if I ever wanted to conceive." I knew I wanted to be a mom someday, and it seemed like this diagnosis had taken my future away from me.

(Hint: I write this as I'm carrying my third child!)

So, I want to tell you a secret: None of the standard implications of PCOS mattered in the long run for me. Through my research and habit implementation, I was able to overcome all standard obstacles women with PCOS face and help thousands of women do the same. Through my one-on-one work and my widely successful online programs, PCOS Boss Academy and Get Pregnant with PCOS, I have seen women from every socioeconomic background make meaningful lifestyle changes that positively impact their daily lives.

WALKING THE WALK

Here's the secret: The key to my community's success is learning how to make our PCOS the North Star of our health. In a way, we are actually lucky because when you have PCOS, your body just has a louder alarm than others. Our bodies have no problem telling us to slowwwww dowwnnn and check up on ourselves. (It just does that through unwanted symptoms like facial hair growth and acne. Smh.)

A missed period, gained weight, or intense mood swings can signal that we must return to baseline, reboot some health habits, and get back on track to be our healthiest selves. The ongoing journey of having PCOS is learning to listen to our bodies, respond compassionately by taking care of our health, and be mindful of how our food and stress affect our hormones and thus our wellness.

What a superpower, am I right? Instead of waiting thirty years to find out we have awful (and preventable) chronic diseases like diabetes, cancer, and high blood pressure (which kill so many people and cause so much suffering), we get to avoid all of that by being on top of our health. Trust me: Our PCOS tummies, hormones, and brains will tell us when we need more veggies, sleep, and sunshine.

So, girl, I promise you, all this effort will pay off eventually. You name the illness—it has a connection to stress and diet. And the top way to manage our condition is by managing our stress and diet. So, how lucky are we that we get to be ahead of the curve and avoid preventable chronic lifestyle diseases?

True, it's not fair that we have to be on our A-game 80 percent of the time (never 100 percent; we are still humans who need burritos). While there is no cure for PCOS—it is a lifetime chronic condition—there are a million ways (and recipes!) to balance your hormones, reduce symptoms, manage your stress, and get back into the driver's seat of your physical and emotional life.

And *that's* what we are going to cover in this book.

Because I have a science and healthcare background, everything I offer in this book is science-backed—no wonky fake news or unqualified internet influencer voodoo up in here. My research on PCOS is supported by what the scientific community has provided as true. And yes, while that might come with limitations (after all, women weren't legally required to be part of clinical research until 1994), we are going with the facts in this book. Not opinions, guesses, or hypotheses. Only what has been *proven* to be helpful.

Managing PCOS is overwhelming enough, and it's time we put a stop to all the misinformation out there.

With that said, here's what's up:

CHAPTER 1
The Not-So-Basic Basics: What We All Should Know About PCOS

The world is complicated, but understanding your PCOS doesn't have to be. Here, we will dive deep into what PCOS is, cover everything the medical community knows about our condition, get clear on the criteria you need to hit to qualify for a diagnosis, and go over the common symptoms most PCOS sisters experience.

Our deep dive into what PCOS looks like doesn't stop there. The reality is that PCOS is like that elusive snowflake: It manifests differently in every single lady. Thus, we will talk about the other lesser-known symptoms that come along for the ride: things like depression, anxiety, fatigue, yeast infections, and body odor. I'll explain why these lesser-known symptoms show up, and later in Chapter Four, I'll explain everything that's in *your* power to reduce these flare-ups.

Finally, we will go over the 101s of getting a PCOS diagnosis, including what labs you need, questions to ask your doctor, and even ways to better advocate for yourself at the doctor's office. And that last part is *not* to be ignored. Hear me roar! Your symptoms are real! You deserve someone who takes you seriously. Let this be the end of any medical gaslighting. All women deserve better. Finally, we'll review how to fire a doctor you aren't vibing with. (Yes, you can do that! BAM!)

CHAPTER 2
What You Didn't Learn in School About the Female Body

Next, we'll learn everything we didn't learn about the female body in sex ed (which is almost everything, ugh). And that means getting up in our female business. That is, up into our vagina.

Knowing about our lady parts—where they are, how they work, and what happens in them—will give you the insight you need to control your flare-ups and elevate your self-advocacy in the doctor's office. You'll be able to ask better questions and, thus, get better answers. After our take on the *Vagina Monologues*, we will cover all things Aunt Flo, ovulation, and the hormones that drive our cycles.

CHAPTER 3
Solving the Mystery of PCOS Symptoms with Science

We will uncover the four main pillars that make up the foundation of your PCOS symptoms: stress, hormones, genetics, and inflammation. Before you sigh in despair, fear not. There is something to do about *each of these pillars*. My recommendations are solution-oriented and don't cost a fortune.

Once we review the steps you can take to decrease stress, support your hormones and genetics, and reduce inflammation, we will dive into what medical doctors describe as "first-line defense," aka the Pill and metformin. I'll tell you a little secret: Those pills are *not* your only option. There are so many other natural ways to level your symptoms and reregulate your ovulation. *Those* choices are centered around nutrition, which we will cover in Chapter Five!

Then, it's time for the real entrée of this PCOS party: symptom mastery through the art of balance.

CHAPTER 4
#Balance: The Art of Finding Balance and Regulating Your Symptoms

In Chapter One, we covered the most common PCOS symptoms, you know, fun sh*t like excessive facial hair growth and weight gain. Well, buckle up because, in Chapter Four, we will get into why these symptoms happen and will create a real science-based action plan for decreasing their potency.

We'll learn how to get that period back on track, keep off those pesky pounds without forgoing pasta forever (Yes! It's really possible!), move toward regular ovulation, and do what everyone told us was impossible: get pregnant naturally.

We will do this by learning we don't have to go keto, become a vegan, or give up bread forever just because we have PCOS. Nah, we can have a diagnosis, keep living our lives, have our cultural preferences and celebrations, plus enjoy cocktails with our friends on Fridays. I promise you, you can have everything you want and enjoy being your healthiest self.

At the end of this section, we'll go over the supplements you need to regulate your symptoms so you can stop adding to that supplement graveyard you may have in the back bottom shelf of your pantry. (Don't worry. I'm guilty, too.) Then, whoa! We're on to Chapter Five—the sweet science of nutrition.

CHAPTER 5
Nitty-Gritty Nutrition

It's no secret what we eat has a huge impact on our health; but do you know how *deep* the rabbit hole goes? All the way down to our gut, plus even farther. What we consume can regulate our blood sugar, prevent diabetes, and get our hormones back on track.

Here, I'll tell you everrrryyything you need to know about food and debunk the myth that eating healthy must break the bank. It's possible to eat good whole foods that aren't million-dollar virgin goji berries washed in unicorn tears only available at Erewhon. Girl, you can get pretty far with just a good ol' tomato.

Then, we're going to get into what's really going to help you: micros, macros, and all the other pieces of the puzzle, like antioxidants and fiber. It's not that hard, and it's not that complicated. By the end of this section, you'll know everything about counting these things.

After we've talked about what you do want to eat, we'll talk about what you don't want in your food. There are some ingredients in processed foods that aren't helping you on your hormone balance journey. We'll also discuss all those "quick fix" diets that are depleting you of nutrients and will only make you run out of steam when you're eating for long-term health. (I'll say it here and a million times over: You do not need to be gluten-free, keto, vegan, paleo, or follow any other restrictive diet to help your PCOS. There is no research that backs this up.)

Boom. After this section, nothing's ever gonna be the same. You'll be able to pick out all the right nutrition info and shut down the diet myths out there.

CHAPTER 6
Supporting Your PCOS

Before we dive into some delicious and great-for-your-hormones recipes, I want to tell you a story about a woman who was able to make all these changes and how much they mattered. After a dark time and some straight-up denial, she finally accepted her diagnosis and got to work. She lost weight, got her period back, and got pregnant naturally with the man of her dreams. We're going to dive deep into the habits that allowed this woman to rock her life, and with her as an example, we'll talk about how you can support your PCOS starting, like, right now. Rebooting your health and achieving long-term success is possible. If she can do it, you can do it.

CHAPTER 7
Things That Taste Good

Now for the fun stuff: recipes! Salty, sweet, savory, zesty—you name it, I have it. We have a six-week meal plan for you that will satisfy any craving and boost your ability to balance your hormones, leaving you feeling full and able to easily and quickly lose weight, if that interests you.

LET'S GOOOOO!

Are you pumped? I know I am! As a registered dietitian who specializes in PCOS *with* PCOS, I know one thing for sure: My history with this diagnosis, my many years battling birth control side effects, weight gain and loss, and my fertility struggles have gone a hell of a long way in cultivating empathy with my patients. My experiences have deeply contributed to my passion for helping others alleviate their symptoms naturally.

After learning and applying everything this book covers, I have seen what I thought would be impossible results. I am stronger, more informed, and a better advocate for my health. When a symptom pops up, I can laugh and say, "Ugh, my PCOS is being a little b*tch today," and not, "I hate my body! It's never going to work the way it should."

So, if you have PCOS and you aren't exactly happy with where you are on that journey, I want you to know you can change direction. And what you need is finally at your fingertips.

My hope for this book is simple: I want you to stop feeling overwhelmed and like you're "different" just because you have this condition. I want you to stop being bounced around from doctor to doctor, feeling hopeless. I want you to see the real, actionable, and sustainable steps you can take to manage your PCOS and live the life of your dreams.

It's possible. I promise.

Even though, yes, PCOS can bring on some sticky obstacles, present big mountains to climb, and give us some problems other girls just don't have, we are in this together. And we can do whatever we set our minds to.

Everything I've outlined here works. I know it works because I've used it on myself to manage my PCOS symptoms for years, keep off almost fifty pounds, get pregnant naturally, and help thousands of women do the same.

And so, after spending years putting all this information together, I want to give it all to you. With the right tools, information, tips, and guidance provided in this book, you can move the needle on your PCOS, feel "normal" again in your body, and let go of the fear that everything is out of your hands. Baby girl, you're in the driver's seat, and I'm sitting right here beside you cheering you on at every turn. Let's get started.

THE NOT-SO-BASIC BASICS

What We All Should Know About PCOS

CASE STUDY ●

Hello . . . Rapid Weight Gain?

At twenty-five, Jordan was rapidly gaining weight.

Twenty-five pounds over three months, to be exact. To her knowledge, nothing—*nada*—about Jordan's lifestyle had changed. Not her diet, exercise, or stress levels. *Except* for the fact that her boyfriend of a few months abruptly left her after the twentieth pound crept in around her waist. That didn't feel too good.

The breakup plus the randomness of the weight gain overwhelmed Jordan. Day after day, she struggled to fit into the stretchiest pants she could find on Amazon. Even XXL wasn't enough. Also,

weirdly, her period randomly vanished. Everything was off. And Jordan had no idea why.

Her body, it seemed, had taken on a life of its own, and she felt like a foreigner in her own skin. After a few months, the ballooning of her hips continued. Jordan was slumped, defeated, and swallowed in sadness. Her self-confidence had never been so low.

Finally, totally at a loss, Jordan made an appointment with her primary care doctor (who was slammed with patients that day). When she walked in, her doctor just glanced at her chart. When it was finally time for Jordan to ask some questions, she stuttered, "But what could cause this?"

Her doctor didn't look up. "Just give up carbs and eat veggies and fish for dinner. You'll be fine. There's nothing really wrong with you."

Then, Jordan's doctor promptly scooted her out the door, and that was that. She got an iced coffee with caramel to cheer herself up and then, at the coffee shop, Jordan started to scroll Instagram.

A reel popped up. It was from a registered PCOS dietitian making a dessert recipe: a cinnamon-roasted peach with Greek yogurt. Then, the dietitian started talking about a condition Jordan had never heard of before—a hormonal condition called PCOS.

Huh? Jordan said to herself. *WTF is that?*

This Instagram lady started to explain what PCOS was and that some of the symptoms could include rapid weight gain and an unpredictable period.

What? Now *that* got Jordan's attention. The more Jordan thought about it, her period had been missing for, like, at least four months (and she for sure wasn't pregnant). And it had been missing since this whole weight gain thing started.

A little idea ballooned in Jordan's head. Maybe, just maybe, she had PCOS,

whatever that was. She clicked Follow for the dietitian's page. After scrolling through recipes, workouts, and information about PCOS—like which medical labs someone should have to be diagnosed properly—a strange and awful thought popped up: *Was she sick?*

Racked with fear and guilt that she somehow gave herself PCOS and her body was just irreparably broken, Jordan booked another doctor's appointment. This time, she brought her phone and showed her doctor the medical lab Instagram reel. At the appointment, Jordan requested those labs. This time, the doctor agreed and ordered a full hormone test and a pelvic ultrasound.

The ultrasound was fast, and it revealed something Jordan had never seen before: a string of pearl-like cysts on her ovaries (a telltale sign of PCOS).

Sh*t.

Then, a week later, the rest of the results were in. The doctor called Jordan and explained she had a high androgen count. This hormonal abnormality, paired with the string of pearls on her ovaries, qualified Jordan for PCOS through the Rotterdam criteria.

. . . .

(The Rotterdam criteria are the three pieces of evidence the medical community requires for a diagnosis of PCOS. The three Rotterdam criteria are: (1) missing or irregular periods, (2) pearl-like cysts on your ovaries, and (3) high androgens, aka male sex hormones, or the physical signs of high androgens like acne or facial hair. This is important if you want to receive a clinical diagnosis for this condition.)

. . . .

"Now what?" Jordan whispered to her doctor on the phone, fear sinking in.

The doctor replied, "Just quit sugar, try to lose some weight, and I'll give you a prescription for the Pill. That will regulate your period. Come back when you're interested in conceiving, because that might be nearly impossible. Have a good day!"

And he hung up.

Jordan was stunned. She didn't have a clue what to do next and wasn't particularly interested in birth control. She grabbed her phone and immediately started scrolling through that dietitian's Instagram for more information. (That page she's on? That's me: Cory Ruth, your PCOS dietitian.)

Jordan binged my content for two weeks before deciding enough was enough. She hired me to be her dietitian, and we went to work.

. . . .

After carefully onboarding Jordan to understand her symptoms and her desired goals, I got her on a high anti-inflammatory diet (think nuts, fish, avocado) and started to carefully observe her cycle through basal body temperature (BBT) tracking, which is a natural way to track your period. (BBT tracking is a tool that uses your body temperature to tell where you are on your cycle. When used consistently, it can be an excellent replacement for birth control.) We followed this protocol for ninety days.

. . . .

Three months later (with Jordan still enjoying tacos with her friends every once in a while), she had lost *all the weight* (plus the five pounds that had been stuck on since, like, forever) and fit into all her clothes again. Her period was back on track, and Jordan had started dating a new boo who supported her PCOS diagnosis like a true gentleman.

Win, girl, win.

GETTING STARTED

It's very possible you read that case study and were vigorously nodding your head.

Me, too, you said to yourself as you read about Jordan's predicament.

Girl . . . same. I know most PCOS warriors were once in Jordan's shoes, myself included. So many of us start our PCOS journey in a similar state of panic and confusion.

When I first got my diagnosis, I was in my early twenties and overwhelmed. And not just because of my PCOS—I didn't even know I had it! I was overwhelmed by the magnitude of being launched into adulthood. I had just graduated school, was saddled with debt, and was crushed by my lack of an answer to the question, *WTF am I going to do with my life?*

The reason I found out I had PCOS was painfully silly. After graduating from college with a sociology degree, I thought I'd make helping people my career, so I signed up for a master's in psychology in San Francisco.

Between you and me, talking about feelings was *not* entirely my forte. But I didn't figure that out for a solid few months. By the time I had decided to quit the program, I had sold my beloved car (the program was in San Francisco! I walked everywhere y'all!). At that point, I was broke, confused, and nearly fifty pounds overweight. My period had been missing for months, I was moody AF, and I had no idea why. (Little did I know the combination of stress with my TBD chronic condition had hit its peak.)

With no clue what to do, I did the only thing available: I moved in with my dad.

This was a little bit out of left field for me because my parents had divorced when I was only seven, and I grew up living with my bad*ss lawyer single mama. But Dad lived closer to SF, and he invited me to stay. Secretly, I was terrified it would go badly, but there was nowhere else to go.

Babes, it turned out to be the best year of my life even though the week I moved in, my dad got a pretty scary diagnosis: prediabetes.

I found out when we went to dinner one night. While we were waiting for the menus, my dad took out his prediabetes testing kit and pricked his finger. Red blood oozed out, and he scooped it up for a sample. He explained to me the science behind the way our bodies use sugar and how too much sugar causes our glucose to spike, and after years of chronically spiked glucose, he had developed insulin resistance, which is what made him prediabetic. And even though I was so sad for my dad, I thought the science behind his condition was pretty cool.

A week after my dad got his prediabetes

diagnosis, my dad's aunt—who had been struggling with type 2 diabetes for *years*—had to be rushed to the emergency room. The doctors announced her diabetes had gone too far. As a result, she had to get her leg amputated.

A couple of days later, we picked her up from the hospital. The poor woman had one less limb than she was born with and looked so weak and frail. I'll never forget how my dad's face fell when he saw the state of his aunt's lower body, bandaged like a wounded veteran.

That evening, I overheard my dad talking to his doctor about what steps he could take to stay healthy despite his diagnosis and avoid what my aunt had gone through. The doctor kept it simple: Diabetes (much like PCOS) has a strong lifestyle and blood sugar component. If you keep your sugar intake low, that will help you keep your blood sugar steady and your symptoms will reduce. Pair that diet change with some stress management and exercise? You'll get better.

My dad was overweight and a total sugar junkie, so I knew that wasn't fun to hear.

But, to my surprise and delight, the next day, my dad turned his life around. He bought a road bicycle and started cycling. He started cooking healthy and cut out all the junk and sugar. In a profound change of events, within six months, my dad completely reversed his prediabetes diagnosis

and lost sixty pounds. We started really enjoying time together in the kitchen, and he taught me so many different cooking techniques. I actually started to like vegetables (a total 180 for me).

Then, my dad bought me a bike. Jobless, I spent the afternoons zipping around the back roads of Sacramento, in between oak trees and cemeteries. It was hot and I started to sweat. Like *really sweat*. It was the first time I had ever done that before, honestly.

Exercise + the fresh veggies + home-cooked meals = I lost a ton of weight.

Girl, I felt so good.

The sudden and profound shedding of fatigue and sadness coupled with the increase in energy got me thinking about a new path—one that would keep me on this new health kick and maybe even help people like my dad and my father's aunt before it was too late. But I wasn't sure what a career in health and wellness looked like.

So, one night, after a cup of fresh spearmint tea with leaves plucked from the garden, I googled *jobs in the health field that require a master's.* I added that last part because I come from a family of doctors and lawyers—my brother is an anesthesiologist—and I always wanted to pursue a higher degree.

On the second page of Google—I know, who even goes there, right?!—I found a blog from a "registered dietitian." *Ring-Ding-Dong!*

I was like, *Oh my gosh, you can work in food and learn the science behind it.* At that moment, I decided I wanted to be a registered dietitian, and the very next day, I signed up to take all the necessary prerequisites at a local community college.

. . . .

Three years later, with all my prerequisite classes—chemistry, biology, anatomy, physiology, microbiology—in check, I applied for a master's degree in nutritional science at California State University and was accepted to the honors program.

That fall, I was knee-deep in *everything* blood sugar and hormones. I learned how nutrition affects every aspect of our health. Moreover, I learned how blood sugar, stress, and hormones are directly influenced by what and how we eat. *Science, it turns out, is important to our wellness.* PCOS wasn't even on my radar yet.

HOW I FOUND OUT ABOUT PCOS

I kid you not, up until my master's program, I had never even heard of polycystic ovary syndrome. That is, until one afternoon, when, as a class, we were reviewing an article that illuminated how PCOS could be treated similarly to diabetes. I did a double-take.

Before I could ask my teacher what it was, my classmate raised her hand and told the class she *had* PCOS! Then she launched into an explanation of classic PCOS symptoms, including missing periods, unexplained weight gain, and hair loss—and how this condition could be treated by stabilizing blood sugar, just like diabetes.

It was like someone threw a bucket of cold water on me. *I had those symptoms.* Unex-plained weight gain. Missing period. It was like she was talking about me. And that was *scary.*

I left the class and went straight to my bed. For a few days, I pushed down my curiosity to read about PCOS. I didn't want to have it. I didn't want to be unhealthy. I didn't want anything to be wrong with me.

That procrastination didn't last long. Because I was in graduate school, I had access to all kinds of scientific articles and journals and had gained the skills of scientific critical analysis to understand them. That Sunday, I opened PubMed (a searchable database of peer-reviewed scientific literature). The more I read about PCOS, the more I was convinced I had it.

You bet I made an appointment with my doc for the next week. I told her about my PCOS hypothesis. After having a full hormone test and waiting a full week, I got my diagnosis. In the wake of my new reality, my doctor said to me, "Cory, you're going to need significant medical intervention if you ever want to get pregnant."

The harshness of her words stuck with me for years. I was truly gutted and I believed her. In this despair, I *spiraled*. Would I never be a mom? Did my body hate me? Why couldn't I be normal?!

My doctor gave me no advice about how to manage PCOS, so I turned to Dr. Google, who effectively told me my life was in grave danger. Everything on the internet was terrifying. Who knew that PCOS greatly increased my risk for type 2 diabetes, metabolic syndrome, endometrial cancer, heart disease, and weight gain? At first glance, this condition seemed like a death sentence.

Moreover, it looked like that doctor was right: It was going to be very difficult—if not impossible—for me to conceive and have a family of my own.

Logically, I figured, since it started in my body, there had to be things I could do to positively influence how my body was responding to this imbalance.

The nerd in me took over. Like a hungry wolf, I tore into every piece of information written about PCOS and read everything about stress, inflammation, genetics, and hormones—the four pillars of this chronic disease—so that I could learn how to master my symptoms and regain control over my life. That research, in so many ways, is the foundation of this book. I want to share all that I've learned so you can take charge of your health and not fall prey to all the misinformation out there.

The more you know about your condition, the more you can take charge of your life and health. I know getting a PCOS diagnosis can feel scary. I know it can feel lonely. But you are in the right place. You are going to learn what you need to learn here to feel less alone, less overwhelmed, and more in control of your life.

And so, we are starting our journey here: learning the basics of what PCOS is, how it manifests, and how you can handle it. My goal with this section is not to depress you, it's to empower you. And with empowerment comes freedom.

THE BASICS: WHAT IS PCOS?

Let's start with the very basics. PCOS stands for polycystic ovary syndrome.

PCOS is a complex condition with a strong lifestyle, endocrine, and metabolic component. It is not curable—no matter what mumbo jumbo that unqualified influencer is telling you. However, your PCOS can be managed by regulating your blood sugar, using food to control your hormones, moving your body, and reducing stress.

Despite the misnomer, PCOS isn't connected to just your ovaries. In fact, it gets its name from the tiny, immature, underdeveloped follicles *on* your ovaries. On an ultrasound, these cysts tend to look like a string of pearls. But here's the kicker: Those PCOS cysts aren't cysts at all! They're actually tiny, underdeveloped follicles that have failed to reach maturity and therefore aren't kicking out your mature eggs. Your PCOS cysts aren't going to burst or cause you pain.

However, your PCOS *could* be behind any fertility issues you may face. After all, it is the leading cause of infertility globally, and it's the most common endocrine condition worldwide. But, ladies, don't let these facts overwhelm you. I offer them to provide per-

spective. Whatever you are going through, you are not alone. One in ten women has this condition.

Although PCOS affects so many women, we aren't taught about it in school. (At least I wasn't!) All I remember from that health class was something about a twenty-eight-day cycle, and *that* ain't true.

But why is PCOS pushed to the sidelines? Well, beyond sociohistorical patriarchal nonsense, PCOS is complicated. It's so confusing that even some medical doctors don't understand it, and that's not entirely the doctor's fault.

Most doctors just aren't trained to specialize in the intersection of endocrine, metabolic, and lifestyle—which is where PCOS lies. Hence, in their confusion, they bounce us around from person to person, hoping we find answers somewhere else. And we just don't. We end up confused, overwhelmed, and stuck.

That stops now. Even though PCOS is complicated, understanding it doesn't have to be. By the end of this chapter, you will understand what this chronic condition is. To help you, I've laid out some basic definitions that will explain the four pillars of this condition.

YOUR BASIC PCOS DEFINITIONS

When you understand the scientific foundations of PCOS, you can ask the right questions to providers and start getting better results. So, let's go over some words and definitions.

WTF Is . . . an Endocrine System?

→ The endocrine system is a messaging system that operates like a feedback loop. The endocrine system's job is to help different parts of our body communicate.

→ What's being carried on this feedback loop is hormones.

→ **Here's how it works:** The main connecting point of the feedback loop is our brain. Our brain needs to communicate with our body. So, the brain sends hormones on the messenger chain. The hormones talk to our glands, and our glands release hormones into our circulatory system (our blood). These hormones land in our organs to be used, and the organs communicate back to the brain with more signaling hormones. That's a very simplified version of the feedback loop. But, basically, one part of our body sends a message to another part of our body, and both react accordingly to the messages being received.

WTF Is . . . a Hormone?

→ A hormone is a super tiny and powerful messenger.

→ A hormone regulates both our physiology (mental health + mood) and below-radar bodily activities (stuff we don't think about, such as digestion, our metabolism, sensory perception, stress, reproduction, and mood).

→ Hormones help regulate how we feel. Some make us want to chill, some make us want to flirt, and some make us super happy.

→ Our environment, regular cycle, and just life can influence which hormones pop up and when.

→ Hormones play a big part in our PCOS journey. When our endocrine system gets out of whack, our body sends all kinds of hormones where they shouldn't be; as a result, our PCOS symptoms increase. That's why when you have more stress, you end up with more hair on your chinny chin chin.

WTF Is . . . Metabolism?

→ Metabolism is how our body converts food into sugar, carbohydrates, and energy.

WTF Is . . . Blood Sugar?

→ Blood sugar is directly related to the metabolic system. Specifically, when we eat a lot of sugar or carbohydrates, our body converts that type of food into glucose. That sugar is sent into our blood.

→ To balance the sugar now pumping through our blood, your pancreas sends the hormone *insulin*. Insulin helps regulate our blood sugar. Think of insulin as glucose's Uber driver—insulin helps shuttle glucose into your cells so you can use it for energy.

→ When our blood sugar is chronically spiked, we develop insulin resistance.

WTF Is . . . Insulin Resistance?

→ When we eat too many carbs/sugar/ starches, eventually our cells stop responding normally to insulin. In other words, the insulin they send to control the party stops working.

→ Too much sugar gives our cells commitment issues. Our insulin ghosts our blood sugar, which leaves glucose hangin' around and causing all kinds of issues like worsened PCOS symptoms and type 2 diabetes.

→ When insulin finally quits, that's when we start to tiptoe into diabetes territory. And this is what we don't want to happen.

It's my opinion that even if we don't work in health, it's important for everyone to understand the basics of how the human body works. While everyone should know this stuff, PCOS ladies definitely need to be aware of how our body functions. After all, each of these things (our hormones, our metabolism, and our blood sugar) plays a significant role in PCOS, and thus, how we can help navigate the complexities of this condition.

Before we dive into how to mitigate your symptoms (Hint: It's largely through lifestyle changes!), you might want to know how to tell if you have PCOS.

And you are about to find out!

SO, HOW DO I KNOW IF I HAVE PCOS?

I hinted at this in the case study, but there are *specific criteria* for getting diagnosed with PCOS. To be diagnosed, you need to meet two out of three of the Rotterdam criteria, which are listed below:

1. Have polycystic ovaries (have "pearls" on your ovaries)

2. Experience irregular or absent ovulation (which shows up as irregular or absent periods)

3. Have excess androgens (aka male sex hormones), identified via labwork or the physical signs of them

Again, you don't have to have all *three* of these conditions to have PCOS. Nope! Just two. *Huh?* you might say. *That's a lot of room for variation for this condition!*

Girl, I know. The trickiest part of PCOS is that there is a ton of room for discrepancy. PCOS tends to show up differently for *everyone!*

My PCOS may look different from that of the woman sitting next to me with PCOS, and *her* PCOS probably won't look similar to the other woman in the room who was just diagnosed. It's a sneaky, elusive little creature, and that's what makes this diagnosis so difficult. For example, here's just one way your diagnosis could turn out: Your ultrasound could have appeared normal, devoid of that classic "string of pearls" look that *all* the textbooks/PCOS websites describe. And guess what?! You may still have PCOS!

Even with no cysts, your period could still be missing and your androgens high—and you can have PCOS.

WHAT CAUSES PCOS?

While the exact cause of PCOS isn't really known, these factors could play a role:

→ **Genetics:** PCOS may be caused by genetic and chemical changes in the womb. Research shows daughters of

mothers with PCOS have a 60 to 70 percent chance of getting PCOS, too.

→ **Hormones:** Hormonal imbalances may be partly to blame. But we're not sure why these hormonal changes occur.

→ **Excess Insulin:** As we covered, insulin is the hormone that's supposed to regulate blood sugar. It is produced in the pancreas, and insulin allows cells to use sugar, your body's primary energy supply. If your cells become resistant to the action of insulin, then your blood sugar levels can rise and your body might produce more insulin. Excess insulin might increase androgen production, causing difficulty with ovulation. Excess androgens are one of the three criteria needed to be diagnosed with PCOS.

→ **Excess Stress:** Oooo. Stress can throw our adrenal glands into overdrive, producing way too much cortisol and DHEA-S (an androgen), which makes our PCOS worse!

While these symptoms all happen internally, they also cause very real external physical and emotional symptoms. And symptoms are what I want to pay attention to next.

THE SYMPTOMS:
KNOWN AND NOT-SO-KNOWN

After treating hundreds of women with PCOS in my virtual practice, The Women's Dietitian, I have gotten an intimate look at the "classic" symptoms of this chronic, lifelong condition. The following are by no means the only symptoms that show up, but they are the most common and the most visible:

→ Irregular or absent period

→ Polycystic ovaries

→ Hair growth on your face or body (aka hirsutism)

→ Hair loss on the head

→ Acne

→ Difficulty losing weight

→ Difficulty getting pregnant

I've always had trouble with irregular periods, mood swings, and hair loss. (This was especially true during times of stress or big life changes! Girl, when I moved in with my dad, I had a full-on bald spot. No fun. No fun at all.)

But these are not the only ways PCOS manifests. There are many other lesser-known symptoms that often go ignored.

After spending years battling my own PCOS issues, helping thousands of fellow warriors manage their symptoms, and deep-diving way too many midnights into PubMed, here are the other symptoms that are hush-hush but oh so present in the daily lives of so many PCOS ladies:

→ Yeast infections (ugh)

→ Anxiety

→ Depression

→ Mood swings

→ Intense cravings (chocolate-covered Cheez-Its, anyone?)

→ Digestion disasters

→ Fatigue

→ Brain fog

→ Body odor

→ Headaches

→ A missing libido

You might be nodding your head to some of these lesser-known symptoms and wondering why no medical professional has ever talked to you about them. Girl, I have my theories. If you are up for it, I want to take a moment and explore my opinion on why these lesser-known symptoms go ignored so often.

PCOS IS A WOMAN'S DISEASE: WHY THAT MATTERS

Fun fact: PCOS is a woman's disease. It doesn't affect men.

That detail is important. To explore and explain why these lesser-known symptoms are rarely discussed and to explain modern medicine's tendency to sweep PCOS (and other women's health issues) under the rug, we need to go back in time. The reason for this systemic overlooking of women's medical issues, at least in my opinion, has much to do with history and the patriarchy.

Long before X-rays and blood tests, before the internet and Instagram, ancient Egyptians wrote records on papyrus that described a peculiar syndrome known as *hysteria*. Hysteria, as a medical condition, was characterized as a manifestation of multiple physical and behavioral dysfunctions. Importantly, it was predominantly a women's issue. Hysteria was a broad term that basically encompassed anything that was out of the ordinary for women.

Soon, a theory emerged: This mysterious disease called hysteria could be the source of most of women's emotional and physical ailments. This idea took hold in ancient Egypt and grew popular. It was so popular that the concept and diagnosis of hysteria trickled down to ancient Greéce and was expanded on by the Athenian philosopher Plato. And Plato was no joke. Plato was one of the geniuses of Western scholarship. But, on top of developing the tenets of Western philosophy (which hold to this day), Plato also produced an interesting medical theory: Female madness could be traced back to a *sad uterus.*

Yup. Plato thought when the female uterus failed to get pregnant, the lack of a baby was the reason women got depressed. The main philosophers of that time, Aristotle and Hippocrates, agreed with this theory and associated the sad uterus with hysteria, the medical condition.

Hippocrates then expanded the origins of hysteria to include an interesting hypothesis: A wandering uterus—on top of being the reason women experienced depression—also wandered through the female body, giving off poisonous toxins to other parts of the body. These toxins would then alter behavior, mood, and health, causing further abnormalities. Ultimately, according to Hippocrates, a wandering uterus was the root cause of various female medical ailments.

Yes. You read that right.

Back in the day, philosophers thought the female uterus would detach and wander around the body, giving off poisonous toxins that made us upset and sick. They also thought that hysteria—a disease that primarily affected women—was the reason we acted out, had depression, or got sick.

While the idea of a migrating uterus was disproven (shocker!), the concept of female hysteria embedded itself in medicine. The idea of hysteria as a *condition* continued to affect future theories, even influencing the godfather of modern psychiatry, Sigmund Freud.

Freud took hysteria to a new level. In 1896, Freud published *The Etiology of History,* where he claimed that the real reason women experienced hysteria was sexual abuse. Thankfully, that was disproven, but Freud continued to say that hysteria was a symptom of *lying* about sexual abuse. When we look back at history, this is when the ideas of hysteria and women lying about their experiences became intertwined.

While Freud's theory was disproved, the idea of hysteria remained strong in the medical community. While hysteria was no longer about wandering uteruses, the idea of the *crazy, exaggerating, lying woman* remained a trope in Western medicine. And it stuck around for a long time. A really long time. The diagnosis of hysterical neurosis was not removed from the *Diagnostic and Statistical Manual of Mental Disorders* (the DSM-III) until 1980. That means, up until 1980, women could legally be diagnosed with hysteria (which was historically associated with women lying or exaggerating about their experiences).

While we all might want to roll our eyes at the ridiculousness of this history, we can't forget about it. It's important because it's the origin of medical gaslighting. Thus, the historical impact of female hysteria as a medical disorder is significant. It has produced generations of practitioners with scientific and/or moral bias, which is more clearly defined as a pseudo-scientific prejudice.

I offer you all this information to prove a single point: The medical community held prejudices against women for a long time, and that prejudice often resulted in women being accused of being hysterical or lying. Historically, the patriarchy used this reasoning to dismiss our medical concerns; unfortunately, the practice of dismissing women continues to this day.

While women's rights and medicine have advanced a ton, this idea of hysteria still lingers in our society. In today's medical offices, women are often still treated as though they are hysterical, and we are still having our symptoms brushed off as our being crazy, or doctors just assume we are exaggerating our symptoms (or even lying).

There's so much research on this, but here are a few examples of how this shows up in contemporary life. A 2018 study found that when men were treated for chronic pain, they were called "brave." But when women were treated for chronic pain, they were labeled "emotional." If we can infer what we've learned about women's history here—that when women felt bad, historically we were given the diagnosis of hysteria—we can see how medical history and past practices are influencing contemporary diagnoses and enabling medical doctors to continue to gaslight female discomfort, pain, and medical issues.

Here's another (all too common) example of women being mishandled and called hysterical: the case of endometriosis. Endometriosis affects *only* women. And it can take six to eleven years to be diagnosed. One of the key factors of this diagnosis delay is that both the doctors (and the female patients) tend to "normalize symptoms." This means that both the doctors and the patients tend to sweep away the pain of endometriosis because they believe that the patients are being hysterical and overreacting to the pain they are feeling. (Since when is it okay that women are in a resting state of pain? Why is that normal? Not in *my* book.) This is just another example of old tropes being applied to modern medicine and patients. Just because something affects only women doesn't mean that we are exaggerating the discomfort we are feeling.

This "normalization of uncomfortable and painful symptoms" persists even when the condition is deadly, like cancer. A 2013 study concluded that *more than twice as many women as men had to make more than three visits* to a primary care doctor in the United Kingdom before getting referred to a specialist for suspected bladder cancer. This is because most women are dismissed for being . . . Guess what? Hysterical. And these delays cause unnecessary deaths. Each year, an estimated *40,000 to 80,000 people die due to diagnostic errors* in the United States alone.

Oy. My point is this: Gender-based medical gaslighting is real, and it's not reserved for just PCOS warriors. But we PCOS ladies feel this pain particularly hard. My clients, myself included, have been made to feel hysterical when we bring our symptoms to our doctors, especially the lesser-known symptoms like depression, anxiety, mood swings, and low libido. Many just don't take us seriously, and we get dismissed or, worse, told it's all in our heads.

I must say this isn't always the case. Many doctors help a lot of people. However, while so many doctors save lives, give life-changing diagnoses, and truly change patients' experiences, there are some (again, not all) doctors who simply refuse to recognize the discomfort women feel. Even though most doctors do their best, this isn't acceptable. Women can't be gaslit or made to feel hysterical when we are dealing with a real medical issue.

For too long, men have written medical books and controlled if and when women can get a legitimate diagnosis. For too long, men decided what pain levels were normal for women. Nah, girlies, all this patriarchal nonsense ends here.

We get to decide if how we feel is good enough.

Ladies, if a doctor has ever minimized your symptoms, made you feel that it was all in your head, or made you feel crazy—I want you to know you are not alone.

And while *it should not happen,* I want you to know that your symptoms—both known and lesser-known—are not in your head. They are happening in your body and have a real effect on your mood and energy levels. You are the only one in your body, and you are the only one who has the authority to tell if your symptoms are real. We can't let history dictate the future of our health. Our symptoms are not in our heads, and they deserve to be treated with respect and legitimacy.

SYMPTOMS

To help you, empower you, and teach you something you may not have known about your PCOS experience, let's dive into the symptoms PCOS warriors face—not just the most common/classic ones. My goal is to show you that, no, your discomfort is not all in your head.

Common (aka Classic) Symptoms

Like I said, there are some cornerstone, classic symptoms of PCOS. While none of these are the root problem of our chronic, lifelong condition, I want to take some time to explore how each of these symptoms is uniquely tied to your PCOS. Understanding how your hormones connect to your PCOS and how your PCOS affects your mood and health will empower you. This knowledge will enable you to finally stop knocking your head against the wall and encourage you to take actionable steps to decrease the potency of your symptoms. (A brief note, however. We are *not* talking about solutions to these symptoms just yet. The solutions come later. For now, I just want to spend some time going over the symptoms, so you know that your pain/discomfort/overall grouchiness is not in your head!)

And so, drum roll, please! Without further ado, here are the most common symptoms.

Irregular or Absent Periods

While there are many reasons your period might be missing, typically the reason you are missing a period is because you aren't ovulating. No ovulation, no period.

(But, babes, if you are reading this book to search for the answer to your missing period, the best advice I can give you is work directly with a professional to determine the cause, because it might be something way more complicated than missing ovulation.) But for now, know that a missing period is a telltale sign of PCOS.

Not Ovulating

While there's a lot of room for vagueness in this field, here's what I know for sure: If you have no period, you definitely aren't ovulating. And PCOS ladies have a hard time ovulating because of how disruptive imbalanced hormones can be. If you aren't ovulating, this is something you *need* to know because ovulation isn't just for makin' babies! Ovulation is a critical reproductive process that is important for every woman regardless of whether the goal is to get pregnant.

Regular ovulation is a sign of happy hormones, and healthy hormone production is an important indicator of good health. So, what is it about ovulation that makes it so special? Aside from being crucial to conceiving naturally, ovulation is the only time we produce a hormone called progesterone. Beyond progesterone production, ovulation is beneficial for:

→ Helping to reduce levels of inflammation in the body.

→ Balancing the powerful effects of estrogen (too much estrogen may cause symptoms of estrogen dominance).

→ Helping prevent health issues like strokes, heart disease, dementia, and breast cancer.

→ Keeping bones strong and healthy.

→ Keeping your metabolism burning (and thus helping your weight loss efforts).

→ Lifting your mood! Progesterone is a very calming hormone.

Every time you ovulate, it is like a deposit into your long-term health savings account. And, of course, you can't get pregnant without ovulating first.

I know you must be asking, "How do you promote regular ovulation?" Well, that's the million-dollar question, and it depends on why your ovulation is not happening in the first place. Here are some common reasons why you might be skipping ovulation:

→ High androgens like testosterone

→ Insulin resistance

→ Undereating

→ Stress

→ Over-exercising

→ Thyroid dysfunction

→ High levels of prolactin

→ Perimenopause

Due to the wide variety of causes for not ovulating, I recommend working with a specialist to get your body back in balance. To determine if you're not ovulating regularly, you can track your temperature via a BBT thermometer along with making an appointment with your doctor's office for a more personalized approach.

Cysts on Your Ovaries

PCOS pearls, anyone?

Having cysts on your ovaries is one of the Rotterdam criteria to be diagnosed with PCOS (along with absent or irregular periods and excess androgens). Again, cysts on your ovaries are the little things that look like your grandma's pearls on ultrasounds.

These cysts are *not* the same thing as the large, heavy, painful cysts that can develop on ovaries and burst or cause pain. Despite sharing a name, ovarian cysts and PCOS cysts are not the same thing at all.

Now, you can have both PCOS *and* painful ovarian cysts—but if you just have PCOS, I want you to know your PCOS does not cause you pain. You cannot feel tiny, immature, underdeveloped follicles!

Abnormal Hair Growth

"Hi, I'd like a beard, please" is something almost no woman would say to her hairstylist.

Yet, so many of my fellow PCOS warriors fight the battle of abnormal hair growth. Some even must shave their face daily after their morning coffee. So, what gives?

Often, high testosterone is to blame. If you have PCOS and your blood sugar runs wild (after eating the standard American diet of Starbucks and fast food), your high insulin levels send messages to your ovaries to pump out more testosterone, and that can cause a whole lot of other problems. (FYI: High testosterone can also cause abnormal hair growth, acne, and male pattern balding.)

Hair Loss

As we've learned, many women with PCOS have elevated testosterone, which leads to symptoms like facial and body hair growth,

acne, hair loss on the head, irregular periods, and weight gain.

If you're noticing more hair shedding and thinning, high testosterone might be the reason. If so, it's time to loosen that ponytail, scoot to the doctor's office, and ask for a lab test. Getting a full hormone panel that evaluates which hormones are high is one of the only concrete ways to establish the root cause of your hair loss. I would also recommend asking the doctor to check your vitamin B_{12}, iron, and vitamin D, as low levels of these can also cause hair loss.

Acne

Me in high school: "Thank God I'll be done with this acne sh*t soon."

My PCOS now: "LMAO, bishhhhh you thought!"

Ugh. It never ends! While so many things could be causing your breakouts, here are a few possibilities:

→ **High Androgens:** High levels of male sex hormones like testosterone and dihydrotestosterone (DHT) may result in breakouts. Lab work can show you if this is a contributing factor.

→ **Diet:** While diet alone won't cause your acne where it otherwise doesn't exist, studies do show dairy (milk, yogurt, cheese) and high-glycemic foods (white rice, donuts, croissants) may worsen acne in those who already struggle with it. This is the only situation where I would recommend a trial dairy elimination for three months to see if it positively impacts your skin.

→ **Certain Skin Products:** Choose products labeled "noncomedogenic" or "won't clog pores." For most, these won't make your skin flare.

→ **Sleeping in Your Makeup:** Even noncomedogenic makeup can aggravate breakouts, so make sure you give your face a scrub before you hit the hay.

→ **Plugged Hair Follicles:** Acne happens when cells close to the surface of your skin block the openings of sebaceous glands and cause oil buildup. Sweat doesn't cause acne, although it's not a bad idea to shower post-workout.

→ **Certain Hormonal Birth Control:** Some types of birth control contain progestins with a high androgen index, which can worsen acne.

→ **Stress:** Although the exact mechanism remains elusive, some research shows stress can exacerbate acne. Prioritizing self-care is critical.

→ **Sharing Makeup Tools:** Acne isn't contagious, but sharing brushes/applicators can transfer acne-causing bacteria, oil,

and dead skin cells to your face, which can clog your pores.

While some of these causes are external (makeup tools, skin care), a lot of what causes acne is *hormonal*. That means you must level out your hormones to see results. The best way to tackle that is through eating for happy hormones.

Difficulty Losing Weight

So many of us with PCOS, myself included, can gain weight like it's our job. It's like all we have to do is look at a piece of food, and the scale goes up ten pounds. There are so many components to weight loss, and PCOS definitely doesn't make this already hard thing any easier. Here are some of my top questions to help you determine if your PCOS is impacting your weight.

ARE YOU STRESSED AF?

Stress can affect your ability to lose weight. Your adrenal glands (which sit right on top of your kidneys like little hats) produce two stress hormones: cortisol and DHEA. Elevated cortisol can slow down our metabolism. When our metabolism slows down, our ability to process foods stalls and our body's desire for sugar and carbs increases. That alone can cause issues with losing weight. DHEA is a similar disruptor, and it can cause problems with ovulation.

ARE YOU TAKING THE RIGHT SUPPLEMENTS?

If your hormones are outta whack (something you need to get tested to confirm), you should be taking supplements to counteract your imbalances. Honestly, my line of supplements, VITA-PCOS, is my answer to all the nonsense sold out there. All my supplement lines are filled with the actual stuff you need to support your PCOS.

ARE YOU EATING ENOUGH PROTEIN AND FIBER?

The truth is what you're eating can make or break your weight journey even if you do not have PCOS. That doesn't mean you have to give up what you love (including gluten and dairy) and go out back to the pasture, munch on grass all day, and be sad. No. It means steadily working toward better blood sugar control with the right macronutrient composition.

DO YOU HAVE A MOVEMENT ROUTINE?

Getting at least thirty minutes of moderate exercise will do wonders for your waistline and mental health. Not moving your body or allowing yourself to decompress and de-stress further drive your hormonal imbalances. Prioritize this.

DO YOU LOVE YOURSELF?

Might sound woo-woo, but if you talk down to yourself, don't believe in your own self-worth, and don't have faith your body can get where it needs to go, this entire wellness journey may be futile. Believe in your own power to change your life. Your body is capable of so much—including healing and being healthy.

Difficulty Getting Pregnant

So, back to the main symptoms of PCOS. Unfortunately, PCOS is the leading cause of infertility globally. Infertility can be a complicated, confusing, and extremely frustrating journey to embark on. But mama-to-be, I am here for you! I've been through hell and back with my diagnosis, and I'm on the other side to teach you how to navigate it all, including getting intentionally knocked up. In fact, I've dedicated my career to the topic.

If you are trying to get pregnant and are struggling, please know you're not alone. There are options (with very high success rates) *besides* expensive fertility treatments to try first. The truth is you might not need any medical intervention to have a baby. Simple changes in diet and lifestyle have the powerful ability to impact our fertility when we have PCOS. Moreover, you don't need to go riding the roller coaster of restriction and eliminate all the things you love to eat to have a baby. We will talk more about practical solutions to infertility in Chapter Four. But for now, know that experiencing infertility is one of the classic symptoms of PCOS.

And that's the last of the "classic" PCOS symptoms.

Before we move on, I want to spend some time illuminating and defining a whole other set of lesser-known symptoms. These symptoms tend to get less attention but are still as prevalent and relevant.

The Lesser-Known Symptoms of PCOS

So many of the lesser-known symptoms associated with PCOS are rarely acknowledged as something a PCOS warrior might experience. Yet, so many of the women I work with tell me they feel these things and, moreover, are overwhelmed by them.

The worst part? My ladies feel alone in their experiences. And isolation feeds depression.

So, I want you to know, as someone who works in the medical field, that these lesser symptoms are not in your head. Your body is legitimately trying to communicate to you that something *isn't* balanced. You are not hysterical.

Your symptoms are real. And there are

steps you can take to move out of this state and into one of balance, mindfulness, wellness, and empowerment. You have full power in your body, life, and mind to rectify that imbalance.

Let's begin with a big one, shall we?

Anxiety and Depression

Women with PCOS are three times more likely to have anxiety and depression. Why? Not only can this be due to hormonal imbalances and blood sugar issues, but it's also *exhausting* to have PCOS.

So, boo, be kind to yourself. Of course, it's hard to try to stay on top of the acne, constant hair loss, and hair growth on our faces and bodies. It's frustrating to feel like you're working so hard to lose weight, only to not see the scale move a pound. And it's draining to feel like we always must eat a certain way when all our friends get to eat whatever they want. Throw in inflammation, insulin resistance, blood sugar issues, and elevations across the hormone board, and then, of course, this disorder seems impossible to beat.

I hear all of this, and I'm right there with you. Please know you aren't alone, love.

If you have acute sadness that just won't go away, you may be wondering what the eff is going on. The exact correlation between PCOS and your anxiety and depression are still hazier than your favorite IPA, but I'm going to break down a few possibilities for you below:

→ Research has shown that women with PCOS may have lower levels of specific neurotransmitters, like serotonin, which help boost our mood and are associated with positive feelings. Women who have these lower levels of serotonin report more symptoms of anxiety and depression.

→ Many women with PCOS have insulin resistance. More research is needed, but several studies have shown people with insulin resistance reported more anxiety and depression symptoms. In addition, blood sugar dysregulation can cause sharp ups and downs in our mood.

→ Finally, this one may be a big duh, but it absolutely deserves a seat at the table. PCOS symptoms can suck. Who wants a period that strikes completely out of the blue (like every time you decide to wear white or have an anniversary) or random chin hairs?! PCOS symptoms are confusing, frustrating, and downright agonizing. They can cause a great deal of stress and sadness, which can manifest as anxiety and depression. *No wonder it's too much sometimes.*

I promise you that when you learn how to manage your symptoms (which you *will* by the end of this book!) and pair that knowledge with nutrition, stress management, and movement, everything will come together. The storm that clouds your mind will soften into a sunset. A future without pressing anxiety and spiraling sadness is possible.

Mood Swings

Again, it's stressful AF to constantly feel like we need to eat like a rabbit just to lose half a pound and to shave our face before work. It's frustrating to feel like we have to restrict the foods we love while our best friends get to eat whatever they want. It's disheartening to feel like we're working so hard and not seeing the results we feel we deserve. That's why more than 60 percent of women diagnosed with PCOS also struggle with their mental health. So, know that you are not alone.

The good news is (and yes, it exists) we can work to lessen the grip our PCOS mood swings may have on us.

One key to navigating mood swings is finding the right supplement routine. For example, taking a cortisol calmer and magnesium supplement can be absolute game changers for many of us who struggle with depression, stress, and anxiety, and I can't recommend them enough!

In short, having PCOS can be overwhelming, but there's so much we can do to lessen the stress and anxiety, and it all begins with lifestyle changes you can make.

Intense Cravings

Why do we get such intense cravings when we have PCOS? It's simple: Because our levels of blood sugar are unstable. When our blood sugar gets low, our bodies crave more sugar and carbs to bring it back up. But the cycle is vicious: Once we eat more sugar, our blood sugar crashes, and we need more sugar and carbs to sustain us. All the while, our insulin (the hormone that regulates our blood sugar) is trying to help our cells drink in that glucose. When there's too much sugar in our blood, insulin can give up. *You had one job, insulin!*

Ugh. What a cycle. So, what can we do? Three words: blood sugar balance.

Managing our mood swings (and weight) is not about calories in, calories out. It's about the right combination of nutrients to keep glucose levels stabilized, in other words, balancing our blood sugar. Balanced blood sugar keeps us fuller for longer, stamps out intense carb/sweet cravings, and regulates our energy levels. *Boom!*

There are other reasons we might be craving pizza, bagels, and nachos. And those reasons are all about our hormones. Here are some basic relationships between hormones and cravings:

→ Elevated insulin and dysregulated blood sugar can intensify cravings.

→ Elevated cortisol (our stress hormone) can make us crave-y AF.

→ Fatigue can be so out of control with PCOS, which can lead us to seek more energy-dense foods to literally fuel us through the day.

→ As we've learned, women with PCOS have higher rates of both anxiety and depression, which can lead many of us to comfort eat! No shame. Really.

The best way to prevent and manage these cravings is to put good food on your plate. Foods filled with protein and fiber (like salmon and veggies with a nice lemon garlic sauce) will keep you fuller longer and help your current (and potentially oncoming) cravings for something like a bowl of mac and cheese or a bag of Doritos.

Fewer PCOS cravings = better chances to reach our PCOS health goals like fewer PCOS symptoms, improved fertility, and easier weight management.

Eating Disorders

The unfortunate truth is, because of how mangled the myths around "ideal" PCOS eating have gotten, many women diagnosed with PCOS also have an eating disorder. I wish it weren't true, but it is.

This sad fact makes sense given all the misinformation out there about what PCOS warriors can eat, can't eat, and how food hits our bodies differently than others.

My darlings, so much of what's out there about PCOS and eating *isn't* true. There is no scientific evidence that you need to be vegan, vegetarian, gluten-free, keto, practicing intermittent fasting or anything else but your perfect self to manage your PCOS symptoms. You don't have to go on a crazy restrictive diet to balance your hormones.

IRL, #balance is the actual thing that will bring your PCOS symptoms to a manageable state. Not becoming a vegan. PSA: It's one of my missions in life to debunk the myth that specific diets help with PCOS. (News flash! They don't. They just drive us crazy and tend to give us an unhealthy relationship with food.)

Digestion Disasters

Believe it or not, PCOS and digestion are intricately connected. When our androgens are high, this influx of hormones can actually make gut health symptoms worse.

Why? Research studies have shown that high androgens lead to a lower diversity of gut bacteria in our microbiome. Our microbiome helps balance hormones, regulates our immune system, digests our food, and manages inflammation. Not only that, studies show the higher the androgens, the lower the gut bacteria diversity is.

Yeast Infections

Since we've learned that PCOS goes all the way down to our gut, it makes sense it goes down farther. In short, PCOS can contribute to yeast infections. Women with PCOS commonly suffer from yeast infections due to imbalanced blood sugar and hormone levels. Effectively, hormonal imbalances linked to imbalanced blood sugar can cause excess sugar to accumulate in urine and set the stage for yeast growth. Uncontrolled sugar levels damage blood vessels and nerves, decreasing lubrication and causing vaginal dryness.

Additionally, birth control tends to shift our natural vaginal flora, so that can also contribute to yeast infections.

Ugh, am I right? Again, balancing your blood sugar can be a great way to mitigate this unpleasant symptom.

Body Odor

Does it ever end? We are almost there with the lesser-known symptoms. This one is definitely one of the least associated with PCOS. It's highly likely your body odor may be tied to your diagnosis.

Body odor is uncomfortable to deal with, and it's extremely frustrating when we can't pinpoint exactly what's causing it! Here are some possible culprits:

→ **Blood Sugar:** Hormonal imbalances linked to poorly controlled glucose levels can cause more perspiration, bacteria, and odors.

→ **Low Estrogen:** Temperature regulation issues associated with low estrogen can lead to hot flashes, which result in more sweating and bacteria growth.

→ **And all those other symptoms (depression, anxiety, mood swings, emotional eating):** Well, it turns out that feeling that way can make us sweat more and, thus, smell worse.

What can be done?

You might have guessed it. You gotta balance your blood sugar! That means eating more whole foods like cucumber, protein, fatty fish, and low-starch veggies.

Headaches

Do you ever get headaches or migraines? If so, there's a good chance PCOS is behind them. From throbbing migraines to persistent tension headaches, I can tell you from personal experience these can be downright exhausting. Like, curl-up-on-the-couch debilitating.

Many of us try to push through and tough them out because we don't want to be perceived as hysterical. We don't want to be crazy, ill, or dramatic, so we ignore the pain away.

Besides, who has time to deal with a headache on top of everything else life throws at us?! Here's why PCOS can be the culprit for these headaches:

→ **Hormone Levels:** When estrogen fluctuates, it can affect the dilation and constriction of blood vessels, leading to headaches. During our ovulation and periods, estrogen levels rise and fall, which is why headaches often occur around periods.

→ **Low Blood Sugar:** When blood sugar levels are low, blood vessels may constrict, causing headaches. Low blood sugar can also trigger the release of stress hormones like adrenaline, which can further contribute to headaches.

→ **Birth Control:** Birth control is a common "solution" for PCOS, but it can also cause headaches in some individuals.

So, myth busted. From estrogen changes to low blood sugar to various methods of birth control, there is a legitimate reason PCOS is causing our headaches.

Still, there are things you can do to help manage them! First, track when they happen so you can identify any triggers. Second, are you getting enough water? Seriously, don't underestimate the value of good ol' H_2O when it comes to headache relief. Finally, are all your supplements languishing in the back of your pantry? Take some out. Supplements like omega-3 fatty acids and magnesium citrate can be so helpful in navigating your headache journey.

Low Libido

Remember when you were young and horny? Oh, the good old days.

Maybe the desire just isn't there, and maybe you just aren't that excited about it. Girl, that makes sense! It's not fun to lose our desire for pleasure and connection.

And that loss might be connected to your PCOS. Why? Along with hormonal imbalances, it can be psychological. Bad body image days, bloat, fatigue, and just the emotional impact of dealing with a chronic condition can be huge contributing factors to a reduced libido in women with PCOS.

Sometimes, a loss of libido can be tied to how we feel about our partners. "Did he forget to take out the trash *again*?" or "I can't believe he had the nerve to say that to my mom in front of me!" Yeah, not feelin' it tonight, sorry.

As I said in the previous section, we need to decrease stress to create a better context to create pleasure. The reason stress interrupts our sexual experience is because during stress, we prioritize survival over everything else, including sex. Our body isn't thinking about having a good time when it thinks there is a threat. It can't distinguish between a life-threatening danger like a predator chasing us and stress that's lingering from your boss yelling at you earlier in the day, so your body is preparing your systems to run from that predator not have an orgasm. The key is to bring your stress to rest, which we'll cover later in the chapter.

Once you've brought down the stress, the best context you can create for having sex, and for having a better orgasm, is one of connection. Everyone is going to have different preferences in the bedroom when it comes to needing foreplay or having sexy music playing in the background. Pay attention to what your body is saying about what it does and doesn't like.

THE POINT

· ·

My intention with this overview was not to depress you but rather to illuminate the very real dark crevices that exist in our medical system. Just because nobody told you these symptoms were going to happen doesn't mean they aren't happening.

If you want concrete evidence for your symptoms, get ya butt to the doctor and get some lab work done. Lab work is one of the best ways to see what imbalances are happening in your body.

LAB WORK

By now, you know PCOS is a sneaky, confusing little thing. It can be overwhelming, inconsistent, and random. One of the best ways to find out what's really up in your biodome is to get medical lab tests done.

Yes, labs can be expensive, but so is spending years trying different diets and different supplement routines and still not getting the results you want. Data is your best friend if you have PCOS. Thus, if it is available to you, I highly recommend getting your labs done.

"But Cory," you may say, "what labs do I get?"

Have no fear! Your trusty dietitian is here to save the day! Below are *all* the labs you need to find out if you have PCOS.

A full hormone panel will usually include, at the bare minimum, estrogen, testosterone, progesterone, and thyroid-stimulating hormone (TSH). Other options you should consider getting tested for are follicle-stimulating hormone (FSH), anti-Müllerian hormone (AMH), luteinizing hormone (LH), dehydroepiandrosterone sulfate (DHEA-S), A1C, fasting insulin/glucose, sex hormone–binding globulin (SHBG), and prolactin.

Here's a bit more info on each of these labs, including why you need them:

FSH (follicle-stimulating hormone)	FSH is a follicle-stimulating hormone. You typically would test that along with LH. Women with PCOS typically have a 2:1 ratio between FSH and LH. If the ratio of LH to FSH is 2:1 or 3:1 (LH being higher), that might indicate PCOS.
AMH (anti-Müllerian hormone)	AMH stands for anti-Müllerian hormone. If you have high AMH, it can be indicative of PCOS. It may also be indicative of ovulatory dysfunction and polycystic ovaries. AMH testing can be done if an ultrasound can't be performed.
DHEA-S	DHEA-S is an androgen produced in the adrenals. High DHEA-S can mean high stress. If your DHEA-S is consistently high, that can indicate that your stress levels could be a driver of your PCOS.

Estradiol	Estradiol is your main estrogen. It is highly involved in the regulation of the female reproductive cycle.
Prolactin	Prolactin is a hormone produced when you're lactating. In some women, elevated prolactin can actually *cause* them to lactate. It can mess up their periods. So, if someone's having irregular periods, we want to rule out elevated prolactin.
SHBG	SHBG is a sex hormone-binding globulin. (No, not goblin!) If someone is experiencing the symptoms of high testosterone, but their testosterone is "normal," I might recommend testing their SHBG. If SHBG is low, there's a chance it's making testosterone *appear* artificially normal or even low.
Fasting insulin test and/or fasting glucose plus A1C (hemoglobin A1C test)	I always recommend getting your fasting insulin test and/or fasting glucose plus your A1C checked. Why? Each can indicate blood sugar dysregulation or insulin resistance. Having these done can confirm if there is some blood sugar dysregulation and/or insulin resistance going on.

Those are the major lab tests you want done. However, if it's available to you, I would also ask for a full thyroid panel. (Some doctors won't do this, but I do recommend finding one who does!) The more data you have, the better.

Here's why: Symptoms of PCOS and hypothyroidism can overlap. Symptoms of hypothyroidism could be weight gain, hair loss, and fatigue. Those could *definitely* be PCOS symptoms, too. So, we should rule out hypothyroidism as being the only issue instead of PCOS. Often, hypothyroidism occurs *alongside* PCOS because it's actually quite common to have PCOS and thyroid issues.

Finally, you can also check on your nutritional status! Iron, zinc, magnesium, and vitamin B_{12} are good ones to check. However, not all these can be ordered at the same time, so be sure to check with your doctor about getting some follow-ups. Also, ask for your vitamin D status. So many PCOS ladies are deficient in vitamin D, which makes us more susceptible to depression and anxiety as well as period irregularities and infertility.

Here's a lab I *wouldn't* get checked: cortisol. If it's super high, you can be diagnosed with Cushing's disease. If it's super low, you can be diagnosed with Addison's disease, but those are two totally separate issues. So, I wouldn't jump to get cortisol tested. I would be looking more at the DHEA-S and the other tests I mentioned above.

HOW TO TALK TO YOUR DOCTOR

Now, if your doctor is less than supportive of running these tests for you, don't give up. You are the patient. You are a paying customer. You are in charge of this dynamic.

You are not hysterical. It's time we step out of the medical stereotype of women, rewrite history, and reclaim our power over our lives and health.

You are experiencing real symptoms and real concerns about your health, and you are (most likely) totally right that something is wrong with you. And you deserve access to the science that will help you figure it out.

Don't get me wrong. There are incredible doctors out there (I've had the pleasure of working with some of them), but being a health practitioner myself, I hear time and time again that women are not feeling heard in the doctor's office. But before we go down a doctor-bashing subreddit—let's stop. Doctors are people who choose a job that helps people. Let's give them the benefit of the doubt that they do want to help you. They just might be swamped with work and their clinic is chronically understaffed.

However, if you find yourself going to the doctor and feeling like you are not being taken seriously, here are three tips to advocate for yourself in a medical setting:

→ Bring a written list of questions. It can be so easy to forget everything we were curious about when we're rushed in a ten-minute appointment.

→ Ask your doctor to please explain your diagnosis, the implications, your treatment options, and all potential side effects of said treatment.

→ If you're just not vibin' with your doc, feel free to switch or ask for a specialist in the issues you're experiencing. If someone does a sh*t job fixing our car, we seek another mechanic, right?! You can switch doctors, too.

If you go to your doctor with your concerns and voice that you believe you might have PCOS, and they *still* won't run labs for you, here's what I would say:

"Understanding what my hormones look like and what they're doing will help inform and guide us into an effective treatment protocol so I can take the right steps to manage my PCOS and health better. I would really appreciate it if we could move forward with my lab work."

Hopefully, after *that*, they say yes to getting your labs done.

If not, darling, you have the right to leave, never go back, and find a new doctor. In fact, if your doctor makes you feel uncomfortable asking for support, I would rather you find a doctor who will listen to you, respond with compassion, and give you useful next steps to manage your PCOS.

If the doctor said yes to ordering your labs—great! However, before you walk out, ask your doctor if you can view their lab order. So often, doctors fail to order all the labs we request, and this leaves us frustrated.

Give them a gentle nudge by ensuring all the labs are requested and thank them for their help.

Again, asking to see your labs isn't pretentious or pushy. You are the patient. You are paying to be there. You have the right to make sure everything gets done.

After you get your labs taken, you play the waiting game. If it comes back positive . . . well, welcome to the club! We eat sweet potatoes and like to party!

YOUR PCOS DIAGNOSIS IS POSITIVE . . . NOW WHAT?

With your PCOS diagnosis in hand, here's what your doctor might say: "Okay, now it's time to lose weight, and you should get on metformin. I'll also give you a prescription for the Pill. Have a nice day. Come back when you want to get pregnant!"

Again, while most doctors do legitimately want to help their patients, this (bad) advice is something I hear all too often. So, I want to spend a few minutes explaining why, exactly, it's so bad.

1. YOU SHOULD LOSE WEIGHT.

Ummm . . . no. Unfortunately, when we have an endocrine and metabolic condition like PCOS, we can't just rely on ol' faithful weight loss recommendations. We have to dig deeper. Simply, losing weight with PCOS is harder. We have a lot of issues other women just don't have. Stuff like insulin, hunger, appetite, and fatigue can make it incredibly hard to reach weight loss goals. So, we can't just follow the formula of calories in, calories out. It's not going to work. Successful weight loss requires getting to the root of hormone imbalance issues.

2. JUST TAKE MEDICATION!

Here's what I think: Taking these medications (like the Pill and metformin) *can* be helpful. At the end of the day, taking medication is a totally personal choice.

However, it's my job to let women know it is not their only choice. Before you jump on the medicine bandwagon, I want you to know that the most often prescribed medication has real potential side effects, like explosive diarrhea, mood swings, and a nonexistent libido. So, there are also real reasons *not* to take them.

If your primary goal is simply to reduce the potency of your symptoms, your best bet is to follow the protocol I will outline in the next few chapters and solve the problem you are facing at its root—not just cover it up with medication.

3. COME BACK WHEN YOU WANT TO GET PREGNANT!

Oh no! No no no! Regulating your hormones, getting your period to come more regularly, and fixing your ovulation is about so much more than just getting pregnant! It's about living in a healthy, regulated body. So, if you are interested in becoming a mama one day, it's better to address everything you need to facilitate a healthy pregnancy now instead of waiting to get your ducks in a row. Basically, the healthier you are, the more likely you are to conceive naturally. So, rebooting your health is a win-win.

MYTH BUSTING

You know what's not true about PCOS? Everything below:

MYTH ONE:
PCOS IS CURABLE.

It's not. PCOS is a chronic, lifelong condition that can only be managed through lifestyle changes, with a heavy emphasis on diet. What you eat has a huge impact on your PCOS, and it is something that we will spend a ton of time on.

Ain't no rest for the wicked.

MYTH TWO:
YOU CAN ONLY BE DIAGNOSED IF YOU FIT THE THREE ROTTERDAM CRITERIA FOR PCOS.

Again, the three Rotterdam criteria are: (1) missing or irregular periods, (2) pearl-like cysts on your ovaries, and (3) high androgen symptoms or high androgens via blood work.

Girl, you only need to hit two of these criteria to be medically diagnosed with PCOS.

And if your symptoms are intense, you've gone to your doctor, and they can't seem to find evidence for your PCOS—go get a second opinion!

No matter what, believe your body. If something doesn't feel right, and you have a gut feeling you have PCOS, you probably do.

You can find the right doctor to help you.

MYTH THREE:

PCOS CAUSES PAIN.

Nope! PCOS doesn't cause pain. Our cysts are not the same ones that burst on ovaries!

There is no scientific evidence that PCOS causes pain, but if you are experiencing pain, I'm not saying it isn't real! Your pain is simply caused by something else, and I would really recommend trying to find out what it is (endometriosis, true ovarian cysts, fibroids, or an infection, to name a few).

THE WRAP-UP

Girl—we went through a lot in this chapter. It took me years of personal struggles, professional research, and hundreds of clinical hours helping patients for me to accumulate this information, so I hope you learned something new about your PCOS.

It's a shame all this information isn't more accessible to the masses—especially considering that one in ten women has PCOS and it is the most common endocrine condition worldwide.

But, we will struggle no longer. In short, here's what we went over:

→ What PCOS is.

→ How to tell if you have it.

→ The vocab you need to know to talk about and understand your condition.

→ The criteria you need to hit to get medically diagnosed with PCOS.

→ What symptoms come along with PCOS (both known and unknown).

→ How the medical history of women relates to that undergirding feeling that our "symptoms are all in our head." They aren't.

→ The labs you need and how to communicate with a doctor to optimize your appointment.

→ What to do if your diagnosis is positive.

The rest of this book is dedicated to helping you live your best life if you have PCOS. And it has to do with lifestyle. The truth? PCOS is a lifestyle condition deeply tied to your hormones and blood sugar, thus, diet and stress management.

When you've mastered these pillars of PCOS, I promise you, you will move mountains. But you need to learn a little more before we get into that.

In this next chapter, we are going to dive into what you should have learned in school about your body. You're gonna get that sex ed class you deserve! We are going to learn all about periods, ovulation, and anatomy so you can be empowered in the doctor's office, ask the right questions, and get the right answers.

Boo, you got this!

No matter what, remember this: You—not your PCOS, not the medical professionals, and not Dr. Google—are in charge of your life. You have all the power, all the tools, and all the smarts to choose your thoughts, take positive action, and move your body toward a healthier future.

WHAT YOU DIDN'T LEARN IN SCHOOL ABOUT THE FEMALE BODY

The Mysterious Case of the Missing Period

Chloe's period was missing. Like, really missing. She wasn't even spotting. After a few weeks, she wondered. After two months, a low-level panic crept in. WTF? Was she pregnant?

After a stressful day at work, Chloe got home, collapsed, stress-ate a few cookies, and then took her butt to the pharmacy. She slinked toward the pregnancy tests, bought a few of them, and went home and did the naughty: peed on the stick.

Anxious butterflies followed by a single, negative line = Not preggo.

What gives?

In the back of her mind, she already knew. Her mom had this thing called PCOS, and she had always struggled with irregular periods. She remembered being warned as a child that it was a potentially genetic condition, but nothing had ever happened to Chloe to prompt her to consider PCOS for herself . . . until her pesky period decided to disappear.

The next day, Chloe called her doctor, went in for an appointment, and told them her hypothesis. Her doctor had seen some PCOS ladies before, agreed that it might be possible, ran a full hormone lab, and did an ultrasound.

Although Chloe's ultrasound came back clean (no pearl-like cysts), her labs were another story. They came back with high androgens. That, paired with her missing period, was enough to qualify her by the Rotterdam criteria for a medical diagnosis of polycystic ovary syndrome.

"Now what?" Chloe said to her doctor when she got the news.

"I honestly don't know much about PCOS," the doctor said. "But, from what I've read, I know there's a huge nutrition and lifestyle component. There are folks who specialize in this. You want to look for a registered dietitian. I'm sorry I can't be of more help!"

Chloe went home and googled PCOS dietitian and found one who offered a course on weight loss and infertility. *Those aren't my problems*, Chloe thought. *But if the dietitian can help with those issues, surely she can help with something as simple as a period.*

Chloe reached out for a one-on-one consultation with the dietitian. (Hint, hint: It's me!) We set up a time to meet, and I had her send me her labs ahead of time. I did an in-depth analysis of her hormone levels before our meeting so that when we talked, we could focus on a game plan.

The day came, and we both popped onto a video chat.

"So," I said, "tell me everything!"

"My periods are missing!" Chloe said. "I haven't had one in, like, four months, and I'm not pregnant. What's going on?"

"Well, I read your lab results, and your testosterone is sky-high," I explained. "So, my first piece of advice is for us to tackle your eating habits so we can get your blood sugar levels under control. That might fix your ovulation, which will positively influence your periods. Still, there are many other reasons your period might be missing. However, before we dive into the science stuff, let me ask you what's going on in your life, stress-wise?"

Then, Chloe started to cry. "My boss is driving me into a corner," she said. "I can't take it anymore! She emails me at 8:00 P.M. and then again at 7:00 A.M. I can't even breathe at work; she shames me for everything I do and then is passive-aggressive whenever I do something *right*. I had, like, four nightmares last night that she murdered me."

"That sounds awful," I said. "That's pretty stressful."

"It is!" Chloe said. "And when I tried to look up what all this stuff was, I had no idea what any of it meant. Like, what's ovulation anyway?"

"I'll teach you all about ovulation, don't

worry," I said. "But beyond the biology stuff, stress *is* a driving force in PCOS symptoms. The stress from your job might have triggered your body to produce too many stress hormones, throwing off your testosterone count. We can get to the root of your missing period with good nutrition, movement, and tackling blood sugar; but girl, you gotta rethink that job!"

"You think so?" Chloe said.

"Definitely."

. . . .

Over the next three months, Chloe and I worked to get her period—and ovulation—back on schedule. In the meantime, Chloe worked with a headhunter to find a new job. She also started tracking her cycle with a BBT thermometer and started eating more of the fab three (protein, fat, and fiber).

By the end of our time together—and with Chloe switching her daily Starbucks and muffin routine to a homemade egg sandwich with spinach and avocado for extra protein—Chloe had made some serious progress! She landed a new job (with a $30K increase in salary!), left that crazy boss, started a new PCOS supplement routine to lower those androgens, treated herself to a monthly Pilates membership, and committed to going three times a week. She even lost a few pounds.

And guess what? Her Aunt Flo came back to visit her every thirty-three days! *Ah-maz-ing.*

. . . .

D id any of that sound familiar? Frankly, Chloe was dealing with a lot, so it's no wonder she was overwhelmed. But her main issue was one that is sadly so familiar: the case of the missing period.

While missing periods are incredibly nuanced and require an individualized plan, for Chloe, her healing experience was all about stressing less, moving more, and tackling her chronically spiked blood sugar. When we focused on these three components for just three months, her period came back.

I know this because I did it for myself. I struggled with having an irregular period for *years* until I got my stress, eating, and movement under control, which I learned by spending countless hours researching. PSA: What I learned about female health during that period of intense research was a game changer when it came to managing my PCOS symptoms.

Schools, society, TV, and magazines all teach us that periods = blood, right? Well actually, periods are only one part of the female cycle, and the other parts of the cycle—follicular phase, ovulation, luteal phase—are super important for our general wellness.

The more you know about your body, the better you'll be able to act against your PCOS symptoms—and that means experiencing less unexpected weight gain, more regular periods, less facial hair growth, and more mood stability. Ready? Me, too.

BASIC BIOLOGY

Pussy Power

First things first, your vagina and vulva are *not* the same thing. Your vulva includes your external organs, like the mons pubis, labia majora and minora, urethra, clitoris, and vagina. Your vagina is actually just the inner canal that connects your uterus to your vulva.

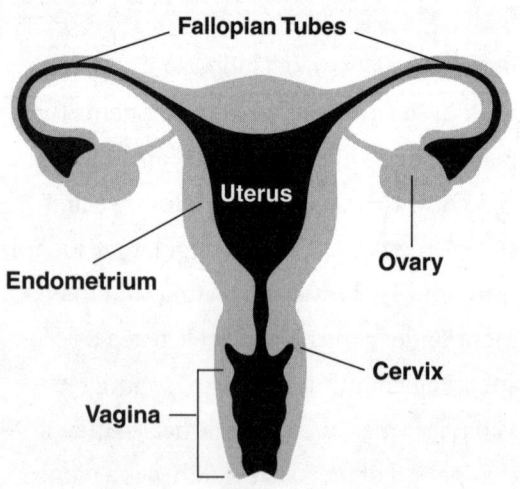

Your vulva is your body's first line of defense to protect the genital tract from infection. When things start to get a little smelly, it's because sweat and moisture might be stuck down there. However, *vaginal odor can also be driven by hormonal imbalances.* If you have some unwanted smells down there, the best thing you can do is not use any fancy washes (they might aggravate the situation more), switch to cotton panties, and reduce your overall sugar intake. Sugar, as we know, can spike your blood sugar, which sends your insulin into a frenzy, and that alone can deregulate your hormones and move your body toward imbalance.

Once you get past your vulva, you'll find your inner labia (your labia looks like lips). Let's start with the facts: All colors of your inner labia are normal. Some inner labia are hairy; some are not. Some women have labia that are asymmetrical, and others are more symmetrical. Puffy, not puffy—it's all organic, baby.

While our cultural preferences (defined by the porn industry) are very narrow, the truth is vulvas are varied and are *always* perfect. If you haven't done a full inspection of your lady bits, I highly recommend grabbing a hand mirror and giving yourself a once-over. Fun and educational.

You'll also find three holes: your urethral opening (pee hole), your vaginal opening (think sex, babies, and blood), and your anus (you know what that's for!).

Get Cliterate

Before we dive into the rest of your anatomy, let's start with the fun stuff: your clitoris. While the penis has four evolutionary purposes (sensation, penetration, ejaculation, and urination), the clit is literally just there to provide profound sensation. It has no other evolutionary purpose than for you to sit back, relax, and enjoy all the calming benefits of orgasms. The clitoris has nearly double the nerve endings found in your average dick. Take that, patriarchy.

Speaking of dicks, one myth I hear a lot—which has been perpetuated by the patriarchy—is that the clit is just a small penis. Umm, *no*. The clit has a totally different anatomy than a penis.

However, both the penis and the clitoris are developed from the same organic material. Here's how: When babies are in utero, it takes six weeks for genitals to develop, and male genitals and female genitals branch off from the same core, developmental cells. Cool, right?

Holla at Your Hymen

The hymen, in my opinion, has gotten way too much attention. While I'm not going to spend a significant amount of time on this, let me just say this about the hymen: There are a lot of myths around this small piece of skin, like it has to be there for a girl to "lose her virginity."

That's a whole lot of nonsense. Some women don't even have a hymen, and if you do have one, it has the potential to heal after it's been broken. The hymen has no biological function, and if you did experience bleeding during an early experience with penetration, it's more likely due to vaginal tearing than your hymen breaking. You don't need to break it to lose your virginity, and your worthiness has nothing to do with the existence of your hymen. Period.

PCOS and Your Vagina

So, how are PCOS and your lady bits connected? As we've learned, hormonal balances influence your whole body, and that includes your vagina.

Our ovaries are where two of the most important female hormones are produced: estrogen and progesterone. When estrogen or progesterone (or both!) are out of balance, the upheaval can throw off your normal menstrual cycle, including bleeding, PMS, and ovulation. When that's paired with high androgens, we can see many unwanted but trademark symptoms of PCOS pop up.

If you have ever experienced recurrent yeast infections, bacterial vaginosis (BV), low libido, vaginal dryness, or even bladder infections, a hormonal imbalance *can be* to blame.

How we fix that is the same advice I will sing over and over forever: Nutrition, movement, and reducing stress levels play a huge role in balancing hormones, especially concerning period irregularities.

How can we support our hormone health? Keep your blood sugar levels steady. Chronic spikes in blood sugar lead to insulin resistance, which throws your hormonal functioning off its regular routine. Over time, chronically spiked blood sugar will lead anyone down the path of diabetes and other cardiovascular diseases (which are the top killers of humans globally!). And PCOS warriors are four times more likely to develop type 2 diabetes than other folks. So even though it's not fair, it serves us best to watch our blood sugar levels more closely than others.

Basically, keeping your blood sugar steady will support happy hormones, regular periods, and ovulation. But let's go a little bit deeper into how all this stuff intersects. Since so many PCOS warriors experience wacky AF periods, let's start with how a period works in the first place. So, my ladies, let's dive into what you never learned in school about your period.

YOUR PERIOD HORMONES

While there are so many hormones in the body, in this chapter, we are going to home in on the hormones that directly impact your cycle. They are progesterone and estrogen.

Progesterone

News and media talk a lot about estrogen, but progesterone is just as important. Think of it as the yin to estrogen's yang. Both have to be balanced for women to experience a normal cycle. A few facts:

→ It's pumped out in the second half of our cycle.

→ Progesterone is our *chill* and *feel-good* hormone that can balance out estrogen levels.

→ Very low levels of this hormone can cause a variety of unwanted symptoms, like anxiety, spotting, headaches, and vaginal dryness.

Mmmkay, you might be thinking, *but what does progesterone do?*

Progesterone has so many vital functions. It thickens our uterine lining, boosts our metabolism, and improves bone health while protecting against bone and endometrial cancers.

Progesterone also acts as a more calming hormone. (When Netflix and an old pair of sweatpants call our name before our period strikes? Thank progesterone.) Progesterone also helps us sleep better! It is so calming that it is even able to relax our bowels. This is why so many of us report digestive issues (diarrhea, constipation, etc.) before our period! (Fun times, I know.)

Moreover, progesterone is essential for maintaining pregnancy, decreasing PMS symptoms, and preventing uterine cancer.

Here's something key about progesterone: *Progesterone is only produced in robust amounts after ovulation.* And that's important. For my ladies who experience irregular periods, you are most likely also experiencing missing/low levels of progesterone.

Or, if you experience frequent spotting before your period or you're finding your cycles getting shorter and shorter, you may be low on progesterone. And if you're never getting a period, you're lacking progesterone altogether.

If any of these symptoms apply to you, it's time to balance your progesterone. Balancing this hormone requires the same commitment to balancing all other hormones: eating well, reducing stress, and moving more.

What About Estrogen?

While estrogen gets hella press, it's not totally unwarranted. Estrogen is super important for our cycle, too. Estrogen gives us all the positive vibes. It can make us Miss Popular, give us our motivating "oomph," and help us get sh*t done! It also boosts our libido and our general desire to be sexual.

Why does estrogen have such an impact on our sex drive? Because, on a biological level, estrogen is essential to ovulation, which is the only natural mechanism that allows us to get pregnant in the first place.

Estrogen also helps us build our uterine lining and protects our bone health. Estrogen is at its peak during the first half of our cycle.

When you have *high* estrogen, you might experience unwanted symptoms like bloating, tender breasts, mood swings, headaches, low sex drive, anxiety/panic attacks, and fatigue.

If you have *low* estrogen, you might experience irregular periods, painful intercourse, depression, memory issues, hot flashes, night sweats, and an increase in bladder infections. (Menopausal women experience many of these symptoms, which makes sense! One of the signs of menopause is a decrease in estrogen levels.)

Whether too low or too high, estrogen impacts all kinds of aspects of our health we might not have otherwise considered. For example:

→ **Weight:** Some forms of estrogen are linked to how the body controls weight. Lower levels of estradiol (the main form of estrogen) can lead to weight gain. Again, we often see this in menopause.

→ **Skin:** Lower estrogen levels are correlated with skin dryness, wrinkling, and thinning. Once skin becomes estrogen deficient, it undergoes histological changes responsible for decreasing collagen.

→ **Libido:** Estrogen helps you feel hot 'n' sexy! This is why you feel your best when estrogen surges through your follicular and ovulation phases.

→ **Energy:** When your body's estrogen levels are out of whack, you may experience major fatigue.

→ **Fertility:** Low estrogen may equal no ovulation, and without ovulation, there is a 0 percent chance of getting pregnant naturally.

How It All Works Together

The best scenario (hormonally speaking) is when progesterone and estrogen both operate at appropriate, balanced levels. While there are a lot of other hormones that impact your PCOS symptoms, we are going to save those for Chapter Three.

YOUR CYCLE EXPLAINED

In this part of the book, we are going to go over how a period works. When you know what a period is and when it's supposed to happen, you'll be better equipped to manage missed periods, regulate ovulation, support your fertility, and get everything back on track.

But here's the truth: Getting a period back on track requires an individualized approach, and I'm not able to provide that level of individualized diagnosis through a book. So, the best advice I can give if you are seriously on the struggle bus with your period is to find individualized support. There are folks out there (like me) who would love to help you.

What I can do for you now is give you a deep dive into everything about your period. Knowing how your period works will empower you to ask the right questions to get the right answers.

The Role of Ovulation

Everyone thinks periods—the shedding of your uterine lining—is the main event of your cycle. It ain't.

The real star of the party is ovulation. Ovulation is a brief period (twelve to forty-eight hours) when your body releases a mature egg. Women are born with all the eggs they will ever have, and those eggs live in our ovaries. Every cycle, your ovaries kick one egg out of the nest, hoping there's sperm out there for it to get a casual drink with. That egg release? *That's ovulation.* The egg is released in hopes of being fertilized.

And even if you ovulate on day 148 of your cycle—you still have a chance at conception. I'll give you a pro tip: If you have PCOS, ovulating every two to three months is perfectly fine.

Remember our hormone progesterone? We only produce progesterone after ovulation. That's important because progesterone is critical to fertility. Without ovulation—

and the progesterone that comes with it—there's no chance of ever getting pregnant naturally. While we will discuss infertility in Chapter Four, know this: If you struggle with infertility, it's not your fault. We learn so much about how to avoid getting pregnant in school, but we never learn how to conceive once we decide to start a family. This isn't right, but it's reality.

Infertility is again one of those situations where I highly recommend patients seek individualized support. Even though you will benefit from specialized support, that doesn't mean you won't benefit from the basics. Getting your nutrition, movement, stress management, and vitamins right will support your fertility journey. I've helped thousands of women conceive naturally through this regimen without expensive hormonal treatments.

But ovulation isn't just for makin' babies, babes! Ovulating will keep our hormones happy, and if our hormones are happy, our body is happy. Ovulation . . .

→ Helps reduce levels of inflammation in the body.

→ Balances the powerful effects of estrogen (too much estrogen may cause symptoms like anxiety, heavy periods, and fatigue, to name a few).

→ Helps prevent health issues like stroke, heart disease, dementia, and breast cancer.

→ Keeps bones strong and healthy.

→ Keeps your metabolism burning (and thus helping to manage weight).

→ Lifts your mood! Progesterone is a very calming hormone.

So, what happens if ovulation doesn't? Point blank: *If you aren't ovulating, your period will go missing.* If your period is coming completely at random or you feel like you're always on it, this is another sign ovulation may not be happening either.

This isn't to say that failing to ovulate is the only explanation for a late period. Things like stress, illness, traveling, thyroid issues, or just plain PCOS could be the culprit for your delayed period or your total lack of visits from Aunt Flo.

Getting ovulation back on track requires a deep look at your eating habits, stress levels, hormone levels, and movement routine. When you get those four pillars moving cohesively, it's more than likely you'll see a return to normal ovulation.

So, What's a Period Anyway?

Before menopause, your uterus has two options: pregnant or not pregnant. When you *aren't* pregnant, your uterus is preparing for pregnancy. A not-pregnant uterus has had its uterine lining built up by progesterone for a whole month. When ovulation happens, an egg is released. If the egg isn't fertilized, it won't become an embryo or implant in the lining of the uterus. Eventually, the uterine lining starts to shed—and you have your period.

To prepare for the next chance of pregnancy, your body must remove all that extra uterine lining. Your period is your body shedding all that lining (which comes out as blood) so it can start again next month.

If your period is off, that means your ovulation is off, which means your hormones are off. And you want to get this back on track ASAP.

The Cycles of Your Cycle

While we all look for blood as an indication of a period, there's so much else going on down there. There are actually four phases of a female cycle. Yes, four!

The first part of your cycle is the menstrual phase.

→ **Duration:** give or take three to seven days on average

→ **Soundtrack:** "Man! I Feel Like a Woman!" by Shania Twain

What goes down: Period day is considered Day 1 of your cycle, or the day Aunt Flo shows up on your doorstep, ready to ruin your favorite lacy underwear. You'll likely feel sluggish and foggy-brained initially, but don't worry—your energy will start to pick up in the next few days as your flow slows and estrogen rises.

On a biological level, when you're bleeding, your uterus is ditching its lining because there's no bun in the oven to cook, so your estrogen and progesterone (key hormones for fertility) levels have dropped. When your uterine lining drops, it comes out as your period blood.

If you've ever experienced cramping, it's because your uterus has been getting swole in the gym for the past thirty days and, as a result, has gained some pretty powerful muscles that are contracting to shed that endometrium lining. Cramping is your body pushing out all the unnecessary tissue.

During this phase, you're likely feeling the continued symptoms of PMS: tired, moody, crampy, bloated, and eating all the chocolate you can find at CVS. And then, like everything in life, it ends.

The second phase is your follicular phase!

→ **Duration:** from the end of menstruation until around Day 14, on average (if you count Day 1 as the day your period started)

→ Soundtrack: "I Feel Good" by James Brown

During your follicular phase, you'll feel your energy rise, your appetite decrease, and your libido skyrocket (thanks, estrogen)! You start to rebuild that endometrium you literally just spent days in agony trying to shed.

You're horny AF because your body is getting ready to release an egg.

What's going on at an emotional and hormonal level during this second phase? Likely, you feel pretty good, have lots of energy, feel social, and are snapping selfies. You can thank rising estrogen for that.

And boom! We are on to phase three: ovulation! This phase is super short but the main event of your cycle.

→ **Duration:** twelve to forty-eight hours

→ **Soundtrack:** "Let's Get It On" by Marvin Gaye

After your period, your hypothalamus (a part of your brain) signals your pituitary gland to send out FSH (follicle-stimulating hormone) to trigger some of your follicles (small sacs of fluid) to get ready, so that one lucky winner can develop into a nice, big, mature egg.

Twenty-four to thirty-six hours before ovulation, LH (luteinizing hormone) surges to signal the release of the egg. That egg will then begin its attempt to get fertilized.

The lonely follicle, now void of its precious egg, becomes a corpus luteum and begins pumping out the hormone progesterone, which will kick off the fourth and final phase.

During ovulation, you'll likely feel friskier than usual. You might notice extra thin or slippery discharge, experience some sharp cramping or a dull, achy feeling, and/or spot a little bit. Thanks to rising testosterone, your libido is at its highest. Boom chicka wow wow.

And just as quickly as ovulation happens, it's over.

Up next is phase four: your luteal phase! This is the time between ovulation and your next period. Progesterone is skyrocketing here. You'll likely feel kinda blah as you get closer to your uterine lining shedding.

→ **Duration:** thirteen to sixteen days on average

→ **Soundtrack:** "Back Up Off Me" by Snoop Dogg

This phase begins the day you ovulate, and you start pumping out progesterone (the hormone that sustains pregnancy). You'll probably feel a little slower, be more prone to Netflix binges, and keep a closer eye on the cookie jar.

There are two options available in the luteal phase. Once you ovulate, if the egg meets a nice, friendly, handsome sperm (one with Michael Phelps swimming skills), your new embryo will travel through one of your Fallopian tubes and make itself right at home in your endometrium. Progesterone will continue to be produced during pregnancy until the placenta takes over the job.

If your egg is *not* fertilized, your egg will disintegrate along with your endometrium and get ready to make its exit via your period, starting the whole cycle all over again. Cue the "Ciiiiiiircle of Life."

Being a woman is complicated. Hormones are strong. Own it, babe. Don't shy away from the dissimilarities of these phases; they are what make us so beautifully unique.

Talk Cervical Mucus to Me

One of the indicators of where you are in your cycle—beyond your mood or bleeding—is the mucus, or cervical fluid, that's coming out of your vulva. Tracking your cervical mucus can optimize your fertility journey and help you understand your own body and where you're at in your cycle! Let's break it down from your least fertile cervical mucus to your most fertile. (Note: Cervical fluid patterns can vary, and this is more of a general breakdown!)

→ **Dry:** This is most common right after your period, and you'll probably feel like the Sahara down there. Fear not, this is normal.

→ **Sticky:** This usually happens during the early and late stages of your cycle, and you'll see white/cloudy discharge that is sticky and often clumpy. This does not facilitate sperm travel. I mean, think about it: Would *you* want to swim through a sea of Elmer's Glue?!

→ **Creamy:** Before and after your fertile window, you'll see thick, creamy/cloudy discharge. This can vary in amount, and it may look like lotion.

→ **Watery:** Right before your fertile window, you'll feel very moist. It's okay, bebe! This clear and wet discharge means fertility is right around the corner. For some of us, this is our most fertile cervical fluid.

→ **Egg White:** Once you see a clear, stretchy discharge that looks identical to egg whites, this is fertile mucus. If you're trying for a baby, it's go time, boo-boo! If you want to avoid pregnancy, better use a backup method like a condom.

The best time to check your cervical mucus is after you go to the bathroom.

Wash your hands and get up in there to see where you fall on the spectrum today.

We Can't Talk About Periods Without Talking About PMS

Girls, we've all been there. Snappy, tired, bloated, boobs swollen, needing *all* the attention and chocolate, and wanting everyone to go away. Welcome to the land of PMS.

About 90 percent of women experience PMS symptoms. But how many of us understand what they are and, more important, what to do about them?

Because PMS is a *problem*. A study found that PMS costs the average American woman $5,000 a year and interferes with work, study, and relationships! No wonder, as PMS includes both physical and emotional symptoms. Feelings include food cravings, bloating, acne, sore boobs, anxiety, depression, fatigue, irritability . . . you name it, it's probably PMS. It can start up to two weeks before your period begins. Cool . . . *not*.

Don't let society fool you into keeping cool about your PMS symptoms. PMS is a very real phenomenon, and it doesn't make you crazy. Female hormones do really dictate how we feel and behave throughout our cycle.

But why does our period affect us so much? Well, when we start our periods, our sex hormones are literally at rock bottom, meaning they've spent the last week or so dropping off. This often means a sharp decline, which can trigger what we know as PMS—so it's not all in our heads. Mood, sleep, libido, digestion, and energy levels are all negatively impacted by these hormone shifts. It's okay if you're not functioning at full speed the day your period shows up. Take it easy and relax, boo. PMS can also get worse in your thirties and forties. This is mostly due to wildly fluctuating hormones like estrogen, which eventually catapult us into perimenopause land.

That being said, should you be crying in pain for days and unable to even look your partner in the eye?! No! That indicates you may have some work to do concerning your hormones.

PCOS AND THE PILL

Oh, the Pill. Let me lead with this: If you want to get or stay on the Pill, I 1,000 percent support that! In my practice, I work with women who are on some form of hormonal birth control, and many (if not most) of them are experiencing some type of sh*tty side effect. The issue *isn't* always the birth control. My issue with the Pill is that our medical community often provides birth control to PCOS warriors to mask our symptoms rather than deal with our root problem: hormonal imbalances.

To date, combined oral contraceptives are the most commonly used treatment modality for PCOS. Why? Birth control pills suppress our androgen levels and replace our natural sex hormones like estrogen and progesterone with synthetic forms, which can regulate bleeding and reduce the symptoms commonly associated with PCOS like acne, irregular periods, and hirsutism. This can tie down our cycle to that classic twenty-eight-day mark.

While hormonal birth control is a convenient and effective contraceptive, it's not for everyone and *it's not designed to balance your hormones or fix your PCOS!* The hormone-like drugs inside them are not the same as the ones our own bodies create.

Yes, hormonal birth control can give us a regular bleed (which is not a real period) and can even clear up acne, but it's doing nothing to get to the root cause or address the underlying imbalances.

When we quit birth control, guess what problems are coming back with a vengeance? *The ones we never addressed before birth control.* And for some women, it can take years to resume normal menstruation after stopping hormonal birth control. This is especially true for women with PCOS.

While I wish there was something simple—like popping a daily pill—we could do to tackle this complex condition, that's just not reality. While I'm not against hormonal birth control by any means, I am in favor of knowledge and addressing the root cause of our problems. If you want to take birth control, that is totally up to you! But before you put anything in your body, you should know what is in it.

If you are desperate to solve your PCOS symptoms, I want you to know that the Pill is not your only option. Personally, it never meshed with me. I experienced some nasty side effects when I was on the Pill throughout college. When I was on birth control, I was never, ever full; I could have eaten a garbage truck full of food, and I would still want fries with that. That appetite change in conjunction with my PCOS resulted in me gaining a ton of weight.

I also experienced really intense (and dramatic) mood swings that negatively impacted my relationship with my college boyfriend (I wish I had known this at the time; the poor guy), on top of increased nausea and decreased libido. At first, I gaslit myself, telling myself I just wasn't normal. But after some time (and getting a medical degree), I realized it wasn't all in my head. Research shows several key nutrients can be depleted while taking hormonal birth control, like vitamin C, B vitamins, magnesium, and zinc. This can potentially affect other aspects of your health negatively, including your energy levels, digestion, and immunity.

I share this with you to let you know that if you can't handle the Pill or just don't like it, there's nothing wrong with you. It was my personal experience and the experience of many of my clients that the side effects were too much.

But this advice isn't for everyone. Some women (like my mother, who's never had a hormonal issue in her life) can take the Pill for decades and never experience any negative reactions. This variation in result (yet again) goes to show how unique all of us are. We must find what works best for us. If you are swallowing the Pill because you think it's your *only* weapon against your battle with PCOS, I want you to know that there are other solutions.

Once I came off the Pill and started eating a nutrient-dense diet and exercising, I lost the weight, and my libido returned. My mood swings resolved, and I didn't get random nausea all the time. Food, exercise, and stress management can be as effective (if not more effective) than the Pill regarding regulating our hormones.

The point of this section is not to dismiss hormonal birth control but rather to highlight potential side effects so you can feel educated and empowered to make your own decisions when it comes to taking birth control.

So, what can you do instead of taking the Pill?

So. Many. Things!

You can track your cycle with a BBT thermometer. (This one is my favorite! I use it to track my period and my ovulation, which helped me get naturally pregnant two times.)

You can also get a full hormone panel done, pay attention to your cervical mucus, and make sure to get a healthcare provider who will help you navigate your symptoms instead of mask them.

What to Do If Your Doc Pushes It?

Unfortunately, it's more than likely that when you get diagnosed with PCOS, your doctor will hand you the Pill, not offer any other advice, and send you on your merry way.

As I've said before, you are your best advocate in the doctor's office, so stand up and ask the hard questions, even when you feel pressured! There should be no "one size fits all" solution. If you need a refresher, here are three tips to advocate for yourself in a medical setting:

→ Ask your doctor for a full lab workup, then ask them to go over all the results with you. Knowing which hormones are out of balance will help you as you try to balance them.

→ Ask your doctor for treatment modalities other than the Pill.

→ If you're just not vibing with your doctor, find a new one who (optimally) specializes in PCOS.

MYTH BUSTING

Here are some myths about the female body that can (and should) be left in the last century.

MYTH ONE:
YOU SHOULD GET YOUR PERIOD EVERY TWENTY-EIGHT DAYS.

Just no. First, let's get one thing straight: If you have an abnormal cycle or don't fall into that perfect twenty-eight-day cycle, don't worry, boo! Less than 15 percent of women have a twenty-eight-day cycle, so stop that shaming if you don't fit into the perfect period box!

MYTH TWO:
BAD PMS SYMPTOMS ARE NORMAL.

While society has taught us to expect extreme PMS (how many memes have we all seen on this?), that's not actually the case. If we are experiencing extreme PMS, we have some level of hormonal imbalance.

MYTH THREE:
OVULATING LATE IN YOUR CYCLE MEANS THE EGG THAT CAME OUT IS NOT FERTILE.

No, girl, no! Even if you ovulate on the one-hundredth day of your cycle, as long as you do ovulate, that egg is just as fertile as someone who ovulates "perfectly" on cycle Day 14. If you ovulate, you have as much of a chance at a healthy pregnancy as the next woman.

MYTH FOUR:
YOU CAN GET PREGNANT AT ANY TIME OF THE MONTH.

Who grew up scared that even *looking* at a boy could get her pregnant? While this paranoia has everything to do with the lack of sex education in this country, the truth is that it's *not that easy* to get knocked up. You only have a small window (the twelve to forty-eight hours of ovulation) for your egg to be fertilized, so only sex during or up to a few days before ovulation can get you pregnant.

THE WRAP-UP

While that's not everything we should have learned in school about our female body—that would be an encyclopedia-size series of books—this chapter aimed to give you a solid understanding of women's health, specifically your period and the hormones that run the show.

Here's a recap:

→ The anatomy of your genitalia! We learned what the difference is between a vulva and a vagina.

→ The power and purpose of a clitoris.

→ How PCOS can affect your pussy. (Hint: It's a strong relationship.)

→ *All* about the two dominant hormones of your cycle: progesterone and estrogen.

→ What ovulation is and how it happens.

→ Some reasons your period might be missing (there are many).

→ The four phases of your period, what happens in each of them, and how they affect your mood, fertility, and libido.

→ Why that b*tchy friend PMS keeps coming over.

→ What the Pill is and what to do if you don't want to take it.

Woo, there you have it: the women's health class we all deserved! The truth is that our PCOS (a woman's disease) can directly impact our female bodies.

Since PCOS is primarily a hormonal imbalance, and our periods are directly linked to our progesterone and estrogen levels, we must support our hormones if we want to reduce unwanted period symptoms or get our period back on track.

While so many other hormones affect our symptoms (and we are diving into those next!), the theme is the same: When we support our hormones, we support our health.

3

SOLVING THE MYSTERY OF PCOS SYMPTOMS WITH SCIENCE

CASE STUDY ·

Facial Hair and the Sh*t Behind It

Jackie wasn't feeling well. Firmly in her mid-thirties, Jackie had always been healthy(ish). After some battles with acne in high school and college, she finally got her skin to a manageable level. But if she had to be honest, all those years sitting at a desk had put pounds on her that her once-a-week jog would not move.

Her annual doctor's appointment was coming up. While she usually just showed up, this time, she had a specific issue she wanted to talk about. Recently, this pesky (and really rather mortifying) problem had been relentless: long, thick hairs growing on her cheeks and chin, along with some gnarly zits. So, when the day for the appointment arrived, Jackie made a point to ask her doctor what could be causing them.

"Hmmm," her doctor said. "Let's run a full hormone panel and find out. Come back in two weeks, and we can review it together."

Two weeks later, Jackie went back to the office. Her doctor stood up, beckoned Jackie over to his computer, and pulled up her chart.

"So, Jackie," he said. "Some things came back abnormal. Your testosterone is unusually high, and so is your blood sugar. In fact, I'm sorry to tell you this, but you are actually very close to being prediabetic. You're a little young for that, so we need to get you on some medication. However, I want to check one more thing before I prescribe you meds. At your appointment, you said you've been having unusual facial hair. Is that right?"

Jackie nodded.

"Okay, then," the doctor said. "If it's okay with you, I'd like to do a quick ultrasound to get a good look at your ovaries."

Jackie nodded again.

"Aha!" the doctor yelled. "Just what I suspected. Do you see these little cysts?" He pointed to the screen. "These are what we call polycystic ovaries—and no, the cysts aren't going to burst, but they do indicate that you have polycystic ovary syndrome. There are a few medications I can give you to help with the overt symptoms—like your acne, body hair, and high blood sugar issues—but, ultimately, this disorder is largely monitored by lifestyle. Others know more about this than I do. You should work with a PCOS dietitian

I can recommend. In the meantime, I'm going to prescribe you something called metformin to help you lower that blood sugar."

In a state of shock, Jackie just nodded again.

While it felt good to have a diagnosis, this was not what she wanted.

After a deep dive into Dr. Google—and *not* contacting the dietitian—Jackie was more than freaked out. PCOS meant that she was *way more likely* to get diabetes, and it was the reason she had so much facial hair. Ick.

Jackie figured she could heal her PCOS with just the medicine. So, she took her metformin prescription religiously . . . and her stomach took the biggest brunt of it: constant diarrhea, bloating, and uncontrollable farting. Talk about adding insult to injury.

Enough was enough. After two months, she quit. Like most women, Jackie was no dummy. She knew she needed to get to her symptoms' root cause if she wanted to see improvements. So, she finally called the dietitian her doctor recommended.

On the phone, I sensed Jackie was scared, frightened. The lack of good information out there had led her to believe PCOS was no better than a death sentence.

But after four months of really focusing

on her blood sugar and upping that run to three times a week, her results were remarkable: Jackie's blood sugar improved, she flipped her prediabetes diagnosis, her testosterone went down, and she saw less hair growth. All without medications that made her live in the bathroom!

WIN!

. . . .

Jackie's story is all too familiar in my book. While Jackie struggled with symptoms, her *real* battle was the straight-up confusion about WTF was going on in her body. Why did she have PCOS? Why was she broken? What was causing her symptoms?

She literally *did not know.*

That's why this chapter is so important to anyone on their own healing journey. With the right information, PCOS doesn't have to be this scary, overwhelming diagnosis. And while, yeah, nobody wants to have a hormonal disorder, this condition is highly treatable. It can even point you toward better health, increased longevity, and a decreased chance of other chronic diseases.

To get all those amazing benefits, we must start with what causes your PCOS. Here, we will cover those four main pillars that comprise the foundation of your PCOS symptoms. They are in no particular order: stress, hormones, genetics, and inflammation.

Before you let the overwhelm knock you out, I promise there is something you can do or some positive action you can take for *each of these pillars.* Most important, none of my science-backed recommendations will break the bank. Because, girl, you are the superhero of your own life. Your superpower doesn't have to be strength or even magical bullet-proof bracelets. Your true superpower is knowledge about what's really going on in your body. With that information, you can make massive changes to your everyday life.

So, if you resonate with any of the case studies in this book and are ready to reduce the symptoms you are experiencing, we must go deep into the root causes of your PCOS. This chapter aims only to illustrate and illuminate how certain factors impact PCOS levels. The next chapter will dive deep into science-based action steps for how to solve them.

One step at a time, ladies, one step at a time!

STRESS

Great topic to start out with, right?

Stress is a huge component in PCOS and basically every other health condition known to woman. It can exacerbate almost anything. The impacts of stress go deeper than you can even imagine. Stress affects virtually every cell in our body.

Now, stress isn't all bad; in fact, the hormones triggered by stress have a biological basis and an evolutionary purpose. But, when left unchecked, chronic stress impacts our immune system and can make us more susceptible to diseases like high blood pressure, diabetes, and ulcers. It affects our mental health, contributing to major physiological disorders like depression. Not to mention, stress affects the quality of sleep we get.

In short, stress impacts almost everything we do and every aspect of our health.

What Is Stress?

Here's a fun fact: There are three different types of stress:

1. **Acute physical stress:** This is when you are literally being chased by a lion, a bear, a tiger, or someone coming down the street. Physical injury or starvation can also cause this. Any of these scenarios will trigger your stress response, but your body is most likely able to manage. Your body will kick your survival instincts into high gear to make sure you don't, well, die.

2. **Chronic physical challenges:** This is your stress response to a sustained disaster like a failed crop season, a long flood, or even a large infestation of bugs. Humans are pretty good at handling these types of long-term challenges. This will still turn on your stress response.

3. **Psychological and social disruptions:** This is where stuff gets interesting. Psychological stress is *all* in our heads. Think about that big fight you had with your mother-in-law. (While it's unlikely y'all would physically come to blows, the situation was still really sh*tty and stressful.)

Psychological stress will trigger the *same biological mechanisms that a chronic physical challenge or acute physical stress will trigger. Your body does not know the difference between psychologically and physically stressful situations.* No matter the type of stress, the same stress response is released in the brain, causing a chain reaction in your cells and muscles.

Here's the major difference, though: Acute physical stress and even longer-term physical challenges *ultimately end*. That is, the injury heals, and the drought subsides. When those experiences end, the body returns to balance. In the scientific community, that balance is called *homeostasis*. The brain has evolved to seek homeostasis.

The problem with psychological stress is that *it never ends*. Thus, when we are inundated with psychological stress, we stay stressed, and our stress cycle never completes. That's why psychological stress is so bad for us.

Okay, cool, you might be thinking. *But thoughts can't be that powerful, can they? They can't literally throw my body into a stress state?*

If you take anything away from this chapter, let it be this: *Even thinking about a future stressful event can tip us toward a stress response.*

Why? Thoughts can trigger the release of certain stress hormones, like cortisol. Cortisol is a little messenger hormone, like Paul Revere on the horse. Instead of shouting, "The British are coming! The British are coming!" cortisol just runs around through our bloodstream, screaming, "EMERGENCY!!! ACT NOW!!!"

That alarm triggers our *stress response*.

So, What Is a Stress Response?

Again, this is a highly simplified version of complex biology, but a stress response is the "rapid mobilization of energy from storage sites and the inhibition of further storage." This means that when you experience stress, your energy—glucose and the simplest forms of proteins and fats—are taken from your cells and redirected to the muscles (like in your legs and arms) that will be used to save you in case you need to attack or run away from a threat.

That's why stress manifests itself physically. Your heart rate, blood pressure, and breathing increase rapidly to transport energy through the body. When your body launches its stress response, your body's priorities begin to shift. This shift is unconscious. You do not control this switch. Your ancient mammalian brain, the one who lived in caves for hundreds of thousands of years, does.

Science calls this switch your *sympathetic nervous system*. When your sympathetic nervous system is triggered, your body stops prioritizing long-term projects like healing, fertility, ovulation, and even digestion. It stops them because these mechanisms are biologically expensive, and *they are not a priority* when you are in a stressful situation. Running away, escaping, and ensuring survival are the priorities.

That's why if you ever get stressed out, you might lose your appetite or feel the sudden urge to poop (or experience constipation). Your body is trying to budget energy for emergencies, so you either need to shed all your excess waste (poop) or shut down your digestive system so energy can be diverted to escaping.

Again, *all that budgeting happens on an unconscious level.*

On the other hand, your conscious behavior—like moving your hand and kissing your lover—is called the *parasympathetic nervous system.* When you are in homeostasis (balanced, calm, in community), your parasympathetic nervous system is the primary control center of your experience.

However, whenever a threat is detected, whether it be physical or psychological, your brain will trigger your sympathetic nervous system and homeostasis is pretty much a lost cause. When serious threats are detected, your brain has two primary modes of protection: fight or flight.

The fight or flight response is very human. It is why, perhaps, when your kids scream at the top of their lungs, you start to scream back (even when you don't want to and it makes you feel like a terrible failure of a mother . . . I speak from personal experience on this one). You yell because you are experiencing stress, and your body wants to use its energy to fight the threat. It is also why, when your boss shames you at work, you have the deep and powerful urge to run away.

When you have these intense feelings as a reaction to a stressful situation, I want you to know there is nothing wrong with you. In fact, you are just a human with a human brain having a human experience. Still, it *is* important to know how you experience stress on a biological level, because serious stress can affect our long-term health.

Here's the truth: Today's issue is *not* the constant threat of being eaten by a lion or even the consequences of a plague of locusts. Can you imagine?!

No, the threat we face today is the *physical and biological consequences of long-term psychological stress.* When we have chronic thoughts that never end and always stress us out, our body *never* gets to reach homeostasis.

When we stay out of homeostasis, our body *always* prioritizes short-term goals (like surviving) over long-term goals (like hormonal balance and ovulation).

Basically, long-term stress is terrible for our health because our bodies never get to focus on sustainable, healthy living. Staying in survival mode wears out our bodies, making us more susceptible to cancer, diabetes, heart attacks, and every other chronic disease out there.

This is bad news, especially for my PCOS ladies.

Stress and PCOS

We know that women with PCOS are three times more likely to experience depression and anxiety than women without PCOS. We also know that we are more susceptible to chronic diseases like type 2 diabetes and heart disease. So what can we do? First, don't demonize any stressful experience. Getting stressed out is normal, and you will experience stress if you are a living, breathing human.

While there is so much complex science behind this—and further research is badly needed—I will break down a few possibilities for how stress is directly related to PCOS. The more you know, the better equipped you will be to prioritize your mental health.

First, having PCOS is inherently stressful. No one wants missed periods, weight gain, or massive zits on their face. Those experiences can trigger shame, and shame triggers stress.

Stress also impacts hormones, which we PCOS ladies are extra sensitive to. When humans are stressed, we have spikes in cortisol. That small hormonal shift can cause us PCOS baddies to experience elevated androgens (male sex hormones). When we experience higher androgens, lots of bad things start to happen: missed periods, weight gain, and facial hair. But what we can count on is

that our insulin resistance increases. When we have insulin resistance, our appetite may shoot through the roof. As a result, we experience intense cravings for carbs and sugar, preventing fat from burning and promoting the growth of fat cells (especially in the abdomen). Cue more weight gain and more stress over (seemingly) uncontrollable pounds.

Stress does more than impact our blood sugar, though. It even has a direct impact on our cycle!

Stress and Our Cycle

Periods and stress are deeply intertwined. I know I'm not the only woman ever to experience a stressful month and have my period vanish. If this has ever happened to you, you might just be experiencing a stress response manifesting as a delayed period.

Why does this happen? Stress, as we've learned, can trigger high cortisol levels, which can disrupt your blood sugar, which can delay ovulation.

On the other hand, a little bit of stress can trigger a different biological avalanche. Your body can start producing cortisol *instead* of pumping out estrogen, progesterone, and testosterone (which we know are vital to optimal ovulation and fertility). This switch causes imbalance, which can result in the classic "my period is late, but I'm not pregnant."

Before you lock yourself in your room and decide to Netflix and chill forever in attempts to avoid all stress, I want to emphasize that what our bodies deem as stressful can look very different. The simple act of jogging for an hour a day or restricting calories may be too much for some of us. The body will register this perceived stress exactly the same no matter what it is, essentially messing up our reproductive hormonal flow.

It totally sucks. All you can do is figure out what is causing you stress, then make small changes to try to manage that stress. I know, I know, that's a big sentence and hard to implement, but the truth is stress is something that is deeply personal and impacts you in the way *that it impacts you*. And stress relief is equally as unique. While I'm not a stress management expert (and I still struggle with this), what you need to know here is that stress is real, and it impacts your hormones and overall wellness.

Just knowing about this correlation is powerful. When you can start to create awareness around what is stressing you out, you can be more conscious about how it affects your life. This awareness is extra important for women who are trying to conceive.

Stress and Fertility

The unfortunate truth is an abnormal hormonal flow can negatively impact fertility.

But, girl, listen, I'll be the last one to tell you to "just relax, and it'll happen." Giant eye roll. But I do have to reiterate the hard truth that stress and fertility are not a good mix.

Again, when we're stressing to the max, our cortisol spikes! This can cause a delay (or a total lack) of ovulation. Because it's 100 percent impossible to get pregnant naturally without ovulation, this can throw a wrench in your baby plans.

To make matters more difficult, to keep a pregnancy once it's achieved, we need progesterone levels to be high. When stressed, our body may favor making cortisol instead of progesterone. That's not good for making babies. Creating environments where our body can prioritize progesterone production instead of cortisol production is crucial if we want to sustain a healthy pregnancy.

If you are struggling to get pregnant, it might be helpful to take an honest look at yourself. If you're working like a dog, doing everything to keep your household running, and stressing over the fact that you're still not pregnant . . . there is a 99 percent chance you are stressed as sh*t. And that won't make the hard journey of fertility any easier.

Stress and the Second Shift

If you manage to have a healthy pregnancy, stress levels do not stop just because you had a baby. No, sister. Take it from me, motherhood is just where the stress begins. Recent studies show women do more than *90 percent of the work in the household.*

(90 PERCENT!!)

Specifically, "women still do the bulk of childcare and domestic work, even in two-earner families in which both parents work full-time and sometimes even when the mother earns more than her partner."

Even more alarmingly, a study found that "men who stood up for their fair share of housework before having kids significantly cut back their contributions after kids—by up to five hours a week."

And that labor shift has major consequences on women's stress levels. "In a survey done by *Today* that interviewed more than 7,000 moms across the country, most moms rated their stress levels at an 8.5 out of 10, mirroring a recent report by the scientific journal *Brain and Behavior* showing women are twice as likely to be affected by anxiety disorders as men."

Babes, the research and numbers are in. Women are so stressed out, overworked, and undervalued that the phenomenon has beckoned a new name: the *second shift.* While so many books and articles have been written about the now infamous second shift, none is more resonant than Eve Rodsky's *Fair Play.*

Fair Play is a new way of looking at household chores, systematizing them, and creating fairness rather than equality between spouses. This system has been praised by many and is long overdue, considering how stressed moms tend to be.

Fair Play doesn't just include physical and visible labor loads (like dishes and laundry). It also includes the *invisible labor* of having a family, like the mental load of having children we don't always think about when we're putting together a cute little pink nursery (and birthday parties, extracurriculars, doctor's appointments, etc.). It also includes the emotional labor of maintaining relationships that come with having a family (teachers, dentists, pediatricians). Acknowledging invisible labor is critical to women's well-being.

Women are so busy that they don't even have time to de-stress and prioritize their own emotional and mental health. In a recent survey by *Healthy Women* and *Working Mother,* 78 percent of moms say "they are so busy maintaining family stability by being constantly available, mentally and physically, to deal with every detail of home life that they aren't taking care of themselves." This is super bad, because if moms can't take care of themselves, they certainly can't do what everyone else expects them to do.

If you resonate with this, you must speak up in your household. The time to end the second shift is *now*. While each family has their own system for organizing their life, if you feel overwhelmed by your share of responsibilities, it's time to acknowledge that your stress levels come first. A new system might be necessary for you to reduce your workload and devote more time to regaining homeostasis (and not mopping).

After all, your health, including your stress levels, is critical to your family's survival. I encourage you to check out *Fair Play* if you are overwhelmed with how to rebalance your home life in a way that brings you and your spouse closer together.

Beyond drowning in laundry—and screaming into the void—here's a little more info on how stress can affect and impact wellness. In fact, you might see a direct correlation between your stress and the prevalence of your lesser-known PCOS symptoms.

Stress Symptoms

Headaches

Remember all the awful lesser-known symptoms we went over in Chapter One? Well, on top of all the regular culprits (high blood sugar, low movement routines, high andro-

gens), stress is also to blame for these random and debilitating symptoms.

That screaming migraine you get every few months? The one that makes even Morgan Freeman's voice sound like nails on a chalkboard? This could happen because stress makes your estrogen fluctuate, and that can affect the dilation and constriction of blood vessels, leading to headaches.

During ovulation and our periods, estrogen levels can rise and fall sharply and quickly, which is why level-five headaches often occur around them.

Stress and Sleep

That eight-hour thing? That's not a joke. Sleeping less than eight hours is not a badge of honor. While the science of sleep is highly complex and specific, here's what you need to know: It's necessary for the health of our brain and body. Sleep is so important that "inadequate sleep—even moderate reductions for just one week—disrupts blood sugar levels so profoundly that you would be classified as pre-diabetic," says Matthew Walker, author of *Why We Sleep: Unlocking the Power of Sleep and Dreams*.

Sleep and stress have a funny, paradoxical relationship. "Not getting enough sleep is a stressor; being stressed makes it harder to sleep," says Robert M. Sapolsky, author of *Why Zebras Don't Get Ulcers*.

So, if you are struggling to sleep because

you are stressed and stressed because you are not sleeping, the best thing you can do is try to break the stress/sleep cycle. Here are some basic steps I recommend.

Consider your caffeine consumption. If you struggle to fall asleep at night, you may need to cut back on your daily cappuccino. I know the haters are going to come at me for this, but science shows caffeine can stay in your system for up to twelve hours, and caffeine consumption can impact your ability to fall asleep later that day.

Beyond keeping you up, here's the thing about coffee: Studies show caffeine increases cortisol (our stress hormone) and epinephrine (aka adrenaline) when resting. After coffee consumption, humans can experience stress levels similar to those experienced during acute stress.

Ah! Who knew, right?

Here's a vicious cycle I see all too often in my practice: A woman has an anxiety attack, can't sleep at night due to caffeine-induced anxiety, feels sluggish in the A.M., downs some coffee to wake up, and the cycle continues. This is not healthy and not helpful.

So, the million-dollar question: Should you quit caffeine? Some people are more sensitive than others, which may be largely due to genetics. If you answer "yes" to any of the following, then my recommendation would *definitely* be to cut back:

→ You have anxiety/feel anxious frequently.

→ You struggle with panic attacks.

→ You consider yourself to have a lot of stress in your life and frequently complain about feeling stressed out.

If you answered yes, perhaps it's time to switch to a gentler option like black or green tea. I'm not saying never enjoy another cup of coffee again (this extremist attitude is so not my style, boo), but if you rely on caffeine every single day and suffer from a lack of sleep and experience chronic anxiety, try switching to a decaf substitute and reserve the real deal for special occasions or days when you seriously need it (y'all know what I'm talking about).

Beyond getting a more balanced relationship with caffeine, here are some more active steps you can take to improve your sleep:

→ **Turn on your blue light filter:** Most phones and laptops have the option to filter blue light and switch to warmer lighting to help you avoid circadian rhythm disruption. You can even set timers so they turn on and off at specific times.

→ **Eat magnesium-rich foods:** Magnesium promotes deep, healthy sleep. Eat more avocados, bananas, almonds, tofu, pumpkin seeds, chard, dark chocolate, and cashews.

→ **Invest in blackout curtains:** Even small amounts of light can disrupt sleep. You'll never go back to the regular kind again!

→ **Establish a bedtime routine:** Train your body to relax in the evening. Try reading a new book, taking a warm bath, lighting a candle, or drinking a cup of chamomile tea.

→ **Make the bed a no-screen zone:** Hard, but so worth it. Other things to do in bed besides scroll: read, have sex, pillow talk, meditate.

Beyond sleep, stress can also affect another thing we all want to be normal and healthy: your weight.

YOUR WEIGHT

Girl, I wish we could get stressed out and eat every M&M in sight without consequences. Or salty potato chips. Or chocolate cake. Or all three. But unfortunately, that's just not the case. What we eat directly affects our health and our weight, especially as PCOS warriors. And our stress levels deeply impact our waistline. Whether we like it or not, the stress and weight connection is real, babes.

As you know, when we're stressed out, cortisol levels can spike. This spike can lead to a big increase in insulin. Big jumps in insulin can cause blood sugar to drop, signaling appetite swings, hunger, and heightened cravings. In addition, high cortisol levels can sloooow our metabolism, which doesn't help with our weight loss efforts.

So, if your heart is set on dropping that extra weight, watch your stress levels.

OUR HORMONES

The next pillar of PCOS is our hormones. By now, we know hormones are key to our mental and physical health. They function as messengers inside the body to regulate your physiology and behavior. They control some of the most important processes in your body, such as your monthly cycle, pregnancy, puberty, menopause, skin complexion, hair growth, fat storage, and muscle loss. We often feel PCOS symptoms the most when our hormones are unbalanced.

When we are experiencing intense symptoms, we tend to feel offff. And that feeling of something not being right is our body telling us that we must focus on our health. However, before we can step into being a wellness hero, we have to figure out what hormones are out of whack. And since no two PCOS warriors are the same, you must get insight into your unique hormone imbalances.

While I've said it before and I'll say it again, getting your lab work done is the best weapon you have to fight and balance out-of-whack hormones. With the data from a full hormone lab test, you can fully evaluate which hormones to rebalance, and that will influence your dietary and lifestyle choices. You should ideally aim to do this roughly every twelve months (if you can).

If going to the doctor isn't an option, you can always opt for an at-home alternative like the DUTCH (Dried Urine Test for Comprehensive Hormones) hormone test, the LetsGetChecked PCOS test, and the GI-MAP (GI Microbial Assay Plus) gut health test. These tests show you what's going on hormonally inside your body and equip you with the data you need to make the changes that matter most. I highly recommend working with a professional to read your results and get a bespoke plan to mitigate your symptoms.

However, after doing this for thousands of women, I can confidently say that getting your hormones back on track starts with proper nutrients, exercise, great sleep, healthy digestion, and reduced stress. That's why I don't put so much emphasis on the type of PCOS, because no matter which type you have, the protocol to heal your symptoms is the same: Eat well, move more, and care for your blood sugar.

While I can't give you a custom plan in this book or give you individual feedback on which hormones are out of balance, I *can* give you insight into how your hormones impact your health.

Stress Hormones

As we've learned, cortisol and adrenaline are our primary stress hormones. Too much of these will increase your body's stress response and, in return, *create more stress hormones!*

Another thing that can impact stress levels is an overactive thyroid. Typically, anxiety is associated with *hyper*thyroidism, and depression is more correlated with *hypo*thyroidism. But bodies are crazy complicated, and this isn't always the case. Regardless, TSH (thyroid-stimulating hormone) levels are directly correlated with anxiety and panic attacks.

Beyond these, synthetic hormones found in birth control also impact mood. A recent study from UCLA found two regions of the brain—the lateral orbitofrontal cortex and posterior cingulate cortex—appeared to be thinner in women on the Pill. These brain regions help us regulate emotions and evaluate our internal state of mind. In women prone to anxiety and depression, hormonal birth control may increase their severity.

I offer this information to you because, in my practice, I often see higher levels of anxiety and depression in women struggling with hormonal imbalances. Because many women with PCOS inherently struggle with hormonal imbalances (it *is* the crux of this disorder), this makes sense. Specifically, I see hormonal imbalances coming from inconsistent or low production of progesterone due to irregular ovulation, lack of a period, or estrogen dominance. It makes sense that the hormone imbalance that would cause low levels of progesterone would also cause anxiety and depression.

Estrogen

Another hormone that directly impacts our PCOS is estrogen. We talked a lot about this in Chapter Two. To recap, poorly balanced estrogen can make us gain weight, lose our libido, increase our risk of mood disorders, and make us feel sooo tired.

This might be the first time you're hearing about how important women's hormones are to our way of life. If it feels overwhelming to you, you're not alone. That's because our patriarchal culture is very much attuned to male hormonal rhythms. Women can never thrive in an environment that wasn't built for us. We are simply built differently. We are basically trying to fit our square peg into a round hole.

If you want to support your estrogen levels, I always recommend you start paying attention to your liver. Your liver is the "cleaner" of your body and is where your body detoxifies estrogen. Yup! This little organ isn't just for helping you out when you drink a little too much tequila (although college me did appreciate the extra TLC). In fact, this organ plays a crucial role in your hormone balance!

If your lab work comes back with high estrogen levels, try reducing the toxins you might be putting into your body (like certain medications, alcohol, or endocrine-disrupting chemicals). You can also incorporate some more cruciferous vegetables like broccoli, cauliflower, and kale to give your liver a little extra lovin'. Leveling this out will only support your hormone-balancing act.

High estrogen isn't the only problem, though; low estrogen levels can cause some frustrating symptoms like low sex drive, weight gain, irregular or absent periods, depression, and painful sex. Ain't nobody got time for all that! Here are some ideas to increase your estrogen levels naturally (without synthetic hormones):

→ **Boost B and D vitamins:** Both of these play an important role in estrogen synthesis.

→ **Chasteberry + black cohosh:** May stimulate estrogen receptors and exhibit estrogenic effects in the body.

→ **Don't undereat fat (or undereat in general!):** Adequate dietary fat and a healthy BMI are crucial for estrogen production. In addition, moderate exercise (not going super hard seven days a week!) will only benefit your plummeting estrogen.

→ **Add more phytoestrogens into your diet (think flaxseed, soy, and sesame seeds!):** Do NOT fear soy! Phytoestrogens have a similar chemical structure to estrogen, but they're vastly different from harmful "xenoestrogens." In fact, multiple studies have associated phytoestrogen intake with decreased cholesterol levels, improved menopausal symptoms, and a lower risk of osteoporosis and certain types of cancer, including breast cancer.

However, estrogen isn't the only hormone that packs a big punch for your health. Androgens (and testosterone is a type of androgen) are the brother hormones to estrogen and directly impacts our PCOS.

Boom! On to the next hormone.

Androgens

Remember what androgens are? They're our male sex hormones, babes! Women make them in the same way men make estrogen—we just typically produce them in smaller amounts than men.

When elevated, androgens increase our risk of insulin resistance, which can increase facial and body hair growth, acne, and our body weight. If you've experienced sudden weight gain and haven't changed much about your diet/exercise habits, it may be worth investigating your androgens and ruling out any blood sugar issues.

High androgens are a very common cause of PCOS symptoms (it is one of the three Rotterdam criteria!).

Probably the most famous androgen of all is testosterone. It's not "just for men," though. Women need sufficient amounts of testosterone, but too much or too little can be problematic.

Insulin

If you ask me, insulin doesn't get enough credit. It's super important for our health.

When you're insulin resistant, your body requires high insulin levels to keep your blood sugars normal. If you have PCOS and your blood sugars run wild (for instance, after eating the standard American diet), your high insulin levels send messages to your ovaries to pump out more testosterone.

This is what could be causing some of your PCOS symptoms like unwanted hair growth, male-patterned hair loss, period irregularities, and weight gain.

Progesterone

While there are so many other hormones we can touch on here, I want to call back an oldie but goodie: progesterone. We know her. We love her. She's an important part of the cycle. All hail progesterone! I'm not going to spend hella time here (cuz we covered her pretty well in the last chapter), but unleveled progesterone can be a major factor in PCOS. It can cause irregular periods, weight gain, and even mood swings!

Gut Health and Hormones

While not a specific type of hormone, I do want to talk about how hormones have a special relationship with our gut. The most popular (and natural) way for our hormones to "talk" to our stomach is through cravings. Hormonal cravings usually sneak up on us when we're PMSing, and they are 100 percent normal. What is not 100 percent normal is when we're having these cravings all day, every day.

Intense cravings can be a sign of a hormonal imbalance or a blood sugar issue. Ultimately, we want to stay mindful of cravings and ensure they don't derail our hormonal health journey (especially important for those of us working on weight management!).

Mindful Product Choices

We can't end the conversation about hormones without discussing endocrine-disrupting chemicals (EDCs). EDCs are primarily synthetic substances in our environment, cleaning products, personal care products, and food sources that may interfere with our endocrine system.

We should care about EDCs because they can potentially disrupt many of our sex hormones, which negatively affect our fertility, hormone balance, weight, and more. One particularly bad—and common—group of EDCs are phthalates, which are used to create faux fragrance in products.

Plastic is also a common one, especially plastics with BPA. There are most likely preservatives like parabens hiding in most (if not all) of the bottles stashed under your bathroom sink, and there is probably BPA lurkin' all up in your Tupperware.

One of the greatest things about the last few years is that the public has become aware of the harmful effects of EDCs, and for-profit companies have come up with economical alternatives. Choosing these alternatives is one of the best ways to limit your exposure to EDCs. Slowly, you can shift your personal care products like shampoo, lotion, and deodorant to more natural versions and toss out your plastic storage containers.

It's far less stressful, money-draining, and overwhelming to replace one item a month than trying to rid your home of all EDCs at once. Try congratulating yourself for your progress instead of beating yourself up for keeping that body butter around a little longer than you'd care to admit.

And finally, remember to be kind to yourself as you try to balance your hormones. It's okay to go slowly. Balancing hormones is never going to be easy, and, unfortunately, it will never be complete. Having PCOS means you have a lifelong condition that requires you to give a little extra effort for your health than most. However, given that most Americans die from very preventable chronic diseases, know that all the steps you are taking to be less stressed, sleep more, and balance your hormones will ultimately promote your longevity.

By implementing the lifestyle changes offered in this book, you will be the healthiest ninety-seven-year-old at the party. Promise.

YOU CAN'T FIX GENES

This chapter is about diving into the four main pillars of PCOS so you can learn what you need to step into a place of empowerment when it comes to PCOS. So far, we've covered stress (a big one) and hormones (another big one), and now it's time for genetics.

Here's the thing about genetics: It's not a fair game, and you get what you get.

And PCOS is one of those things some of us may wish we had never gotten. The exact etiology of PCOS is still largely unknown, but we do know there is a big genetic link.

Women whose moms have PCOS are approximately 60 to 70 percent more likely to have a PCOS phenotype.

While you didn't cause your PCOS and you can't control whether you give it to your daughter, there are habits you can adopt that will empower you to manage your health—and your daughter's health—if this condition eventually comes her way. Over years of trial and error, I finally learned that lifestyle choices can and do impact PCOS. While genetics are powerful, so are habits.

If you have a daughter and you have PCOS, I hope this book helps you sleep a little more soundly at night because, should she have it, too, you have the unique honor of passing down all your knowledge to her. Now that's a bad*ss mama right there. Cheers to that!

And while PCOS can suck, it has become my superpower and boosted my health in many unforeseen ways. It allowed me to invest in long-term solutions rather than short-term fixes.

I can't tell you how good it felt and how much my whole perspective and world changed once I shifted how I was looking at managing my PCOS to one of abundance rather than scarcity. I am healthier than I ever would have been without it.

You can be, too. And so can your children (or future children). Healthy habits can be a family tradition, and we can solidify those as solid as any DNA.

And although PCOS has no cure, we can absolutely manage this beast effectively. With that said, let's tackle the last pillar of PCOS: inflammation.

Inflammation

Inflammation is one of those words in my book that has lost its emphasis. But what is inflammation really?

Normally, inflammation is your body's natural defense against injury and infection. When we experience these injuries or infections, our body sends out chemicals and white blood cells to take care of the job. (That, although simple, is what inflammation is.) Once those injuries are healed, the inflammation is supposed to stop. With chronic inflammation, however, the chemicals and inflammatory cells are always there.

This leads to symptoms like joint pain, skin issues, swelling, fatigue, and headaches. Chronic inflammation even makes you prone to infection and depressive symptoms. It can happen all over the body, causing swelling in not just your joints, but in your organs, too, which puts you at risk for other conditions like heart disease. And as always, the body lives in a loop: Chronic inflammation can worsen your insulin resistance and contribute to weight gain.

Everything seems to cause inflammation, and everything seems to be heightened by inflammation. While this is—to an extent—true, here we will examine inflammation through the lens of PCOS.

PCOS is complex. It entails significant clinical implications for reproductive health, metabolic health, adverse cardiovascular risk, and a greatly increased chance of depression and anxiety. So, it makes sense that inflammation undergirds the root cause of the diverse and somewhat diabolical symptoms this disorder can throw at us warriors.

Inflammation and PCOS

Research shows women with PCOS have elevated markers of inflammation and are chronically in a state of low-grade inflammation. How do you know if you are suffering from high levels of inflammation? Well, thankfully (or not thankfully), inflammation can manifest itself as physical sensations.

If you are experiencing PCOS symptoms along with fatigue, IBS, small intestinal bacterial overgrowth (SIBO), headaches, joint pain, and chronic skin conditions such as eczema, you may have inflammation.

But what causes inflammation? While the true scientific answer is vague and complicated, anything out of the ordinary can cause inflammation. Inflammation can manifest in increased white blood cells, which throw off the body's efforts to fight irregularities, wounds, and illnesses.

PCOS ladies are more susceptible to inflammation because our bodies have a low tolerance for sugar (that's why metformin is so often prescribed to us).

The Snowball Effect of Inflammation

What we eat may trigger inflammation, and inflammation can directly stimulate the production of excess ovarian androgens, which we know may contribute to unwanted symptoms. Research shows that hyperandrogenism can also be the cause of low-grade inflammation and may cause insulin resistance, which can, in turn, further stimulate off-balance hormones and increase PCOS symptoms.

Thus, the snowball effect is both awful and clear: PCOS can cause inflammation, and inflammation can increase the likelihood of PCOS, making patients more likely to suffer from unwanted symptoms like insulin resistance, diabetes, and obesity.

Ahh! What's a girl to do? Don't worry; we are going to dive into the steps you can take to decrease inflammation in the next chapter, but for now, we are going to focus on what you don't want to consume.

What You Don't Want to Consume

What we eat clearly has an impact on our inflammation levels, but what we choose to avoid also has a massive impact on our health. While I will preach balance to the ends of this earth, there's one thing that, any way you look at it, is bad for you: smoking. I could spend a million pages explaining why, but effectively, the smoke you are inhaling causes all sorts of deadly illnesses like cancer and chronic inflammation.

If you do smoke and you have PCOS, quitting will support your journey to rebalance your inflammation and hormone levels.

And we gotta talk about drinking. There is lots of confusing information out there on drinking, especially when it comes to red wine (which has antioxidants). While the conversation on health and alcohol will surely continue to the end of time, here's what science shows to be true.

Even a little alcohol can harm your health. Excessive alcohol use can contribute to chronic conditions like liver disease, can-

cer, heart disease, and inflammation. The current US dietary guidelines recommend no more than one glass of alcohol per day for women. Anything above that is considered excessive use of alcohol. And that one glass a day isn't intended to be averaged over a week. If you don't drink anything during the week and then you have three glasses of wine at dinner on Saturday, that's *still* excessive consumption.

Why are the rules so stringent?

Well, alcohol is quite poisonous to the human body. When you drink alcohol, the booze gets transformed into acetaldehyde, a chemical toxic to human cells. Acetaldehyde damages DNA, which creates an environment more suitable for cancer tumors and prevents the human body from healing.

Thus, if you want to start a new journey with your inflammation levels, one of the first steps you can take is to control what you don't consume, and that can start with stopping your cigarette habits and cutting down your alcohol intake.

Also, girlies, ultraprocessed foods like baked goods, chips, bread, and fried foods do not help your inflammation. While they might taste great, these types of foods are high in refined sugar, simple carbs, and trans fats. They are fine in moderation, but too much of these foods can spike insulin resistance and increase inflammation.

Pills, Pills, Pills

We already know some doctors might not always give the best PCOS advice. Again, that's not entirely their fault. PCOS is a lifestyle and dietary condition; most doctors get approximately one nutrition class throughout their entire medical school journey. One! They also spend their *entire* education learning about how medicine works, so when PCOS warriors come to them with problems, they offer medicine! Shocking, yes?

We've already learned how and why they offer hormonal birth control as a method to regulate hormones—and why that is not your only option to level your unwanted symptoms.

However, in my personal experience and after spending more than five years helping women regulate their health naturally, there is another type of medicine I see prescribed to PCOS ladies regularly: metformin. Or maybe you've heard about inositol. And I know you'll be curious about GLP-1s like Ozempic and how they might help with PCOS.

Let's talk about 'em.

Metformin

Currently, metformin is the most commonly used medication for diabetes, and it is the third-most prescribed medication in the United States, with more than 92 million prescriptions in 2020.

Metformin was first described in scientific literature in 1922 (so we've known about it for more than one hundred years!) by Emil Werner and James Bell. It wasn't until 1957 that France introduced the medicine, and Americans adopted it in 1995.

Metformin's power comes from its ability to decrease glucose production in the liver and to increase insulin sensitivity throughout the body. It also helps lower androgens (a high count of androgens can contribute to PCOS symptoms). As we know, regulating hormones can be a powerful tool in ovulation and, thus, pregnancy. To date, metformin has had positive effects on women attempting to conceive by helping them regulate their ovulation and weight.

However, metformin also comes with some potentially nasty side effects: diarrhea, intense nausea, and abdominal pain.

Many of my clients come to me because they are desperate for these side effects to stop. So, I want to take a moment to point out that the desired effects of metformin (lowered glucose production and increased insulin sensitivity) can be *naturally accomplished* through food and lifestyle choices! Taking these active steps will also naturally increase your fertility.

We can decrease our glucose levels by consuming less processed sugar; eating less processed sugar will naturally decrease insulin resistance. This shift in eating can accomplish the same effects as taking the medication. And eating a well-balanced diet doesn't come with any nasty side effects. (Just the opposite: I think you'll probably have more energy and a slimmer waistline.)

GLP-1s (aka Ozempic)

This is a second drug your doctor may have recommended if you've been diagnosed with diabetes or your weight is really bogging you down.

Ozempic, aka semaglutide, can be injected once a week to help your pancreas regulate its release of insulin. It used to be prescribed only for type 2 diabetes, but doctors are prescribing it for weight management now because of how much weight patients are losing on it.

Like every medication, Ozempic can have some side effects: nausea, constipation, acid reflux, too low blood sugar, and feeling really tired to name a few. These are usually temporary, though, and can be addressed through a variety of tactics.

Taking something like Ozempic is entirely up to you, but here's what I DO want to say on the subject: Changing your food and lifestyle choices while on the medication can help increase its effectiveness, reduce certain side effects, and help you maintain your weight loss should you choose to discontinue it.

Maintaining these diet and lifestyle changes can be a more permanent solution to your insulin and weight loss issues. Metformin and Ozempic, while they undeniably can be helpful, will unfortunately only work on their own for as long as you take them.

Inositol

My favorite natural alternative to metformin and Ozempic is inositol. Here's how it's different: Inositol is a supplement made from vitamin B_8, while metformin and Ozempic are prescription-only drugs. Inositol basically does the same thing as metformin without the annoying side effects—and they can actually be taken together.

I always suggest talking to your doc about inositol if you're having negative reactions to metformin. But don't just follow the doctor's orders. The most important thing when taking medication is to listen to your body. Your body will communicate with you about what's helping and what's potentially hurting you.

While there are limited studies on inositol, current studies have found a huge improvement in conception, ovulation, and weight management while on inositol. Inositol can also help lower androgens, and you don't even need to go to a doctor to renew.

MYTH BUSTING

MYTH ONE:

I NEED TO KNOW MY PCOS TYPE!

Not really. While getting data about your condition is the most powerful thing you can do to treat your unique PCOS snowflake, ultimately, I find people put too much emphasis on finding out their "type." In reality, the end result is the same: To treat your symptoms, you must balance your stress levels, sleep better, eat well-balanced foods, and move more. No matter which type you have, these core active steps will help you reduce your symptoms.

MYTH TWO:

BEING STRESSED ALL THE TIME MEANS I'M JUST REALLY PRODUCTIVE AND A GO-GETTER!

Nope, nope, nope. Being stressed for a long period of time is really bad for you, girl. It's bad for your body, prevents your tissues from healing, and can even harm your fertility. While our society prioritizes work over rest and encourages women to work that dreaded second shift after we come home from work, we must take active steps to reduce our stress levels. Whether that means talking to our partner about the redistribution of chores or just taking a nightly bubble bath, anything you do to rest and de-stress will help your health.

MYTH THREE:

I SHOULD JUST TAKE METFORMIN IF I HAVE HIGH BLOOD SUGAR.

You can, but it's not your only option. While metformin can decrease your blood sugar and increase insulin levels, you can tackle your diet and add some inositol and get better results. The key? Again: PFF! (Protein! Fat! Fiber!) and a little bit more movement can work wonders.

THE WRAP-UP

You can return to this chapter again and again for information/inspiration when you are facing hard times. After all, information about the root cause of your PCOS is your greatest weapon for overcoming your symptoms, getting your health back on track, and living peacefully with this chronic (and incurable) condition. Understanding—and not masking—the root causes of your PCOS will get you the best, longest results.

If you're anxious to learn how to treat these issues, the next chapter is everything. We are going to review all the symptoms and review my science-based action plan to solve them! After the next chapter, your unwanted symptoms are gonna go poof! And girl, you'll thank me later.

#BALANCE

The Art of Finding Balance and Regulating Your Symptoms

Infertility, Who?

Kira knew her clock was ticking. At thirty-nine, it was like her chance to have a baby was disappearing as fast as the hours of the day. She wasn't always this way. In fact, Kira spent most of her twenties declaring she would be the fun aunt forever and, thus, had been on a steady stream of birth control since she was eighteen. While her doctor had told her a long time ago that she had a thing called PCOS, Kira never worried about it because she was already on the Pill.

Then one day, when she was thirty-six and single AF, everything changed. Kira was at a coffee shop when she suddenly remembered she left the stove on.

In a flurry, she put her phone on the table and rushed out the door. Thankfully, her apartment was only a block away. When she got home, her stove was off. Exhausted from the adrenaline rush, Kira reached for her phone. Then, feeling the empty space inside her jacket, her heart skipped a beat. Her phone wasn't in her pocket. So, just as fast as she ran to her apartment, she sprinted back to the coffee shop.

As she ran inside, she stumbled, falling

to her knees in front of, of course, a really cute dude with a nice smile. He looked down at her. "Whoa! You okay?"

His name was David.

While she never got her phone back, she did get a boyfriend.

. . . .

I met Kira and David a few months after they were married, and they decided they wanted to have a family together. Kira knew PCOS complicated fertility, but she didn't have any time to waste. Her goals were to get off the Pill and get pregnant. All in a year.

And girl, we got to work.

For three months, Kira and I focused on redoing her diet and supplement regimen to increase nutrient intake that supported egg quality. We homed in on antioxidants, anti-inflammatories, and nutrient-dense whole foods.

And because it takes two to tango, Kira got David on a similar diet.

We also focused on movement. To get Kira on a more intentional movement routine, Kira signed up for a walking club. Beyond getting in her steps, this club brought some new friends who were in the same phase of life as she was. The community helped her stress level a lot.

Within six months, Kira was pregnant, and all without significant medical inter-vention. Actually, with NO medical inter-vention at all.

BOO-YA!

Kira's success isn't super special (no of-fense, Kira).

Over the years of working with clients, I've had hundreds of women achieve con-ception naturally. Some of those women had even gone through hundreds of thou-sands of dollars of IVF procedures with no luck. Yet, after working with me for just a few months, they got pregnant. Wow, right?

This goes to show that any PCOS symp-tom can be overcome with the right plan in place, even the really sticky stuff, like weight loss and infertility. Despite what doctors might say, there are ways to com-bat these obstacles naturally.

That's what we are going to dive into here: how to naturally (and scientifically) decrease the most potent symptoms of PCOS like infertility and weight gain.

Since so many of the symptoms PCOS warriors face are caused by a handful of hormonal imbalances, we are going to work backward here. I will review the pri-mary *causes* of symptoms (high testoster-one, low vitamin D, adrenal dysfunction) and then explain which imbalances cause these symptoms.

I am doing this because PCOS mani-fests so differently in every lady that it would be impossible to list all the symptoms and science-based action plans for them. Instead, I want to focus on the root cause of these symptoms and explain what actionable steps can be taken to address them so that you can have real results. By looking at the root causes of the symptoms, you will get the most insight into your particular set of issues and get a hands-on look at what you (my special lady) need to work on.

After all this, I am going to take your hormonal regulation game to a whole new level: We dive into the mystery of the supplement drawer. We will finally lay out a plan for which supplements you should be taking based on what symptoms you experience. No more digging around Whole Foods for random stuff. Nah, girl, we will get specific in your quest for healing. Yes, PCOS is a real pain in the butt, but managing it doesn't have to be.

THE ROLE OF DATA

All my information, advice, and protocols are backed by *science*. Science is the best methodology we have to combat PCOS symptoms. Since science starts with data, your healing journey should start with it, too. Here is the data you should be collecting:

→ Your labs

→ Your cycle

→ Your sleep

→ Your calories and macros

Each piece of info will give you insight into your unique body. Your labs can be done with a doctor or through an at-home test like the DUTCH test or the LetsGetChecked PCOS Test (for more on these tests, see page 77).

I love my BBT tracker for my cycle, I like to track my sleep with my phone, and I love to check in and see what my diet looks like calorie-wise and macro-wise on different apps.

When you start to keep track of these stats, you are more likely to find the culprit behind your symptoms. With that said, let's dive into the root causes of PCOS symptoms and what science has taught us we can do about them.

High Androgen Levels

Elevated androgens are a b*tch. Irregular levels of these hormones, like testosterone and DHT, can cause many of the symptoms that throw a wrench in your quality of life. We went over how it could be the culprit behind irregular periods, abnormal hair growth, acne, male pattern balding, and difficulty losing weight.

So, what's a girl to do?!

First, get tested! Get annual lab tests from your doctor to find out if you suffer from high androgens in the first place. There's no reason to go solving a problem you don't even have.

The Solution

Say your lab data illustrates that you have high levels of testosterone. If that's the case, there are ways to balance this out naturally.

First, supplements are a great place to start. You'll want to take a mix of:

→ Zinc

→ Saw palmetto extract

→ Stinging nettle

→ L-alanine

→ L-glutamine acid

→ L-glycine

→ Pine bark extract

→ Inositol

(If you're looking for a supplement to help lower androgens, my PCOS supplements have some of the best androgen blockers on the market.)

Other solutions can include incorporating two or three cups a day of spearmint tea. This is proven to lower testosterone levels. I have a spearmint plant in my garden, which is a low-maintenance, high-reward houseplant. If you have some space and sunshine, I recommend planting one and using the leaves as tea all year long!

If you have high DHEA-S (another androgen, except this one is produced mostly in your adrenals), your body may be overreacting to stress. This can cause symptoms like mood swings, poor sleep, and crazy wacky periods. Try some of these supplements:

→ Phosphatidylserine

→ Ashwagandha

→ Rhodiola

→ L-theanine

→ Magnesium

This, along with really prioritizing stress reduction and high-quality sleep, can help bring down this number. But do you want to know an expert tip? Androgen levels are particularly sensitive to sugar.

When your blood sugar is high (for example, when you are eating a lot of processed candy/bread/pasta/sweets), those chemicals send your body on a roller-coaster ride. That up and down causes your brain to tell your ovaries to pump out more androgens, which fuels symptoms like acne, weight gain, and irregular periods.

So, if you want to level your hormones, first level your blood sugar and steady your insulin levels.

Insulin Resistance

While we are here, let's talk about insulin. Many PCOS ladies struggle with insulin resistance and the different issues it causes. Wacky blood sugar levels can contribute to inflammation and estrogen excess, which is why we may get sore breasts, super painful cramps, fibroids, or even a crime scene flow! So many of our root causes of PCOS come from imbalanced blood sugar. Like, basically every single one.

If you've learned one thing so far about PCOS, it's that it is a lot like diabetes, meaning that it is a metabolic condition highly correlated and sensitive to our blood sugar levels. So, we PCOS warriors must be extra mindful of the special relationship we have with blood sugar and our sugar intake. Chronically spiking our blood sugar will lead to insulin resistance, which, in time, will build into a diabetes condition. We don't want that! Diabetes can lead to cardiovascu-

lar disease, chronic kidney disease, limb amputations, and even stroke.

The Solution

Because PCOS looks different on everyone, what works for the woman with PCOS next to you might not work for you. However, balancing insulin is something we can all undertake.

One of the best ways to even out your insulin is to find the right balance of nutrients for your body. Eating a diet heavy in protein, fat, and fiber will make all the difference in how you look and feel. However, this doesn't mean giving up carbs and sugar forever.

Balancing insulin is all about being mindful of our food intake because, ultimately, the foods we eat affect our blood sugar levels. No matter what we eat, our blood sugars affect our hormone levels. And our hormone levels have a direct impact on how well (or how sh*tty) our PCOS is behaving.

Eating less sugar and fewer carbs will result in more stable blood sugar levels, which decrease insulin and reduce male hormone levels. Eating a PFF (Protein! Fat! Fiber!) diet will support your insulin in controlling your glucose. The magic of PFF is that even if you eat carbs, PFF will help naturally negate a blood sugar spike.

Low Vitamin D

The next issue I see across the board with PCOS ladies is low vitamin D levels. Being deficient in vitamin D can cause many problems, like hair loss, irregular periods, fatigue, depression, anxiety, and other symptoms we associate with seasonal depressive disorder. I mean, have you ever gotten out of bed, looked out the window, and seen only gray clouds on the horizon? Then, did you crawl right back into bed and not get out again for, like, a little too long?

Well, babe, you might be vitamin D deficient. And if you have PCOS, bets are that you are chronically low in this much-needed vitamin.

The Solution

The number one natural source of vitamin D is as organic as it gets: the sun.

Here's how that exchange works. Effectively, your skin has a type of cholesterol that acts as a transformation agent for sun rays. When the sun hits your skin, the rays hit your skin's cholesterol, and that combination of forces allows the body to take in vitamin D.

Science shows that sun-derived vitamin D may circulate in the body twice as long as vitamin D from food or supplements. Fifteen to twenty minutes of direct sunlight will help you raise your vitamin D levels (but

don't forget to put on sunscreen!). And remember, we can actually still get vitamin D on cloudy days, so don't avoid getting outside just because the sun isn't beaming!

How much vitamin D do you need? Well, there's a lot of debate about that. While there are a lot of different numbers out there, the National Academy of Medicine suggests 4,000 IU of vitamin D. If you are in a place that is dark for long periods of time, I highly recommend getting on a regular vitamin D supplement.

If you are super sad, however, and you are getting enough sun, you might just be extra stressed.

Stress and Adrenal Dysfunction

After Chapter Three, you are basically a stress expert. Chronic, never-ending stress, as we've learned, is detrimental to your health. It creates a condition in your body that literally shifts your hormonal flow from its steadfast, balanced, tried-and-true routine of making ample progesterone to making a whole lot of cortisol. This shift is bad for your mental and physical health. And we know too much cortisol causes unwanted PCOS symptoms.

On top of that hormonal shift, stress makes your serotonin too low and your oxytocin (our bonding hormone) too high.

Stress basically throws everything off and makes your PCOS symptoms much wilder and more unbearable.

But the truth is stress is a normal part of the human experience. No matter who you are—I don't care if you are Queen Goop herself—if you are a human, you are going to feel stressed. (So don't get stressed about being stressed, 'kay?)

The Solution

So many books, experts, and resources are devoted to helping people manage their stress levels. While I am not an expert in this field, I would highly recommend *Burnout* (2019) by Emily Nagoski, PhD, and Amelia Nagoski, DMA. This brilliant book illuminates the science behind completing the stress cycle so people can more easily move in and out of the stress cycle and spend more time in homeostasis.

From my own experience—and the research in *Burnout* backs me up—the best way to combat the stress cycle is to exercise. I always say that if someone could figure out how to put one hour of a good aerobic workout—like jogging, swimming, cycling, walking, gardening, or dancing—into a pill, that pill would be the most powerful antidepressant in the world.

So, sweat it out, girl! When you sweat, you are literally running from that "lion" (which may very well be thoughts about your upcoming wedding). That movement and the endorphins running through you are telling your body you are safe!

But don't feel like you need to go hard at the gym seven days a week for hours on end! In fact, going this hard and doing too many high-intensity workouts may lead to unwanted cortisol spikes and cause insulin resistance to get worse. Instead, aim for gentle exercises you enjoy, but keep them consistent!

Exercise will also help your PCOS. Sweating from aerobic exercise has been proven to be an effective way to prevent breast cancer, constipation, insulin resistance, prediabetes, type 2 diabetes, and so much more. Moreover, there is overwhelming evidence that exercise leads to a longer, healthier lifespan.

Exercise is not the only solution to stress. If you suffer from intense stress, don't underestimate the importance of good-quality deep sleep—aim for at least eight hours per night. Try to get to bed and wake up at the same or at least a similar time to encourage a healthy sleep routine.

However, if you are trapped in a chronic, physiological stress response, even a lot of exercise and attempts at sleep won't make a mark on your body's constant release of cortisol and adrenaline.

If this is the case, you'll have to change your lifestyle to support your stress levels. If it means changing your job or moving to a calmer environment, consider what you can do. I know it's scary to make a big change and *not* live the life everyone expected you to live, but if it means reducing your stress levels, your entire body will thank you.

Finally, prioritize self-care. Easier said than done but absolutely critical when your cortisol is soaring sky-high. Most important, what you choose to do to care for yourself doesn't have to be expensive.

I used to think self-care was only for the Hollywood uber-wealthy. It ain't. Self-care is picking—and committing—to an activity that calms you. It can be journaling, hiking, yoga, a hot bath, a warm cup of tea . . . all of these are great options to explore and will help in your journey to minimize stress and reduce its impact on your life.

What matters most is that you have the insight and tools to manage that stress and bring your body back to homeostasis at a reasonable pace. Having a consistent self-care routine is critical for this. It doesn't matter if you spend a million dollars on weekly massages or have a four-dollar face mask from Walmart that you love; with some self-care, your body will move toward completing the stress cycle.

Additionally, supplements such as magnesium, adaptogen herbs, and vitamin D may be helpful to alleviate your symptoms of intense stress, calm your adrenals, and help you feel better.

Finally, what we eat (or avoid!) can play a large role in regulating our anxiety. Magnesium, tryptophan, probiotics, and vitamin B_6 are incredibly powerful nutrients for reducing anxiety. Here are some sources of these anxiety-reducing nutrients.

Magnesium	Almonds, spinach, cashews, avocados, dark chocolate, bananas, pumpkin seeds
Tryptophan	Milk, chicken, salmon, sesame seeds
Foods high in probiotics	Kimchi, tempeh, kombucha, miso, kefir, natto
Vitamin B_6	Bananas, salmon, chickpeas, potatoes, green beans, turkey, carrots, sunflower seeds

My most important tip of all is cheesy AF: Remember to be kind to yourself. The world is hard enough without you shaming yourself for being stressed.

Inflammation

The next "root problem" of PCOS is inflammation. Women with PCOS are more likely to experience chronic inflammation and consistently show higher levels of inflammatory markers. This means we have to be extra mindful of how inflammation can affect us. Inflammation may cause or exacerbate PCOS symptoms like insulin resistance, weight gain, fatigue, headaches, and mood disorders. Whether we like it or not, we have to deal with the inflammation elephant in the room.

The Solution

One of the primary, science-backed ways to combat inflammation is to eat a low-inflammatory diet. Studies show that women who eat a low-glycemic diet (foods rich in omega-3 fatty acids and low in sugar) see positive results when it comes to reduced inflammation and weight levels.

Omega-3 fatty acids reduce inflammation in your intestines and colon. It's a natural lubricant for smooth and gentle elimination. Eating enough omega-3s will help you take regular poops if that's something that interests you. (My personal motto is take no sh*t, but take good sh*ts.) Fish is a great source of omega-3s, but if you don't like fish, fish oil supplements are a great alternative.

I'm going to go out on a limb and say you probably already know you should eat more omega-3 fatty acids. You've probably heard every influencer telling you to eat more fish, avocados, and nuts (and avoid candy and saturated fats).

And yes, to an extent, they are right. But I will tell you a secret: Your body needs some saturated fats. And you, as a human, will want some sugar.

So, if you've decided that you want to take on the battle of reducing your inflammation—

congratulations! Every person can stand to take that step. (Given the state of our environment, EDCs, and the standard American diet, everyone could reduce their rates of inflammation and be better for it.) However, you don't need to eat seven almonds every two hours (or whatever that silly rule is) to decrease your inflammation. You can do so by following a balanced diet that contains a heavier load of fish, nuts, turmeric, and ginger and eating enough PFF. It can be that simple.

Eating a diet that decreases inflammation will support your PCOS journey. It will be the domino effect that can tip your hormone count toward balance rather than disbalance, so you can see the decrease in unwanted symptoms naturally.

Beyond eating omega-3s, eating antioxidants—a type of vitamin found in plants and fruits—can help reduce inflammation. Power punchers vitamins C and E are some of the most notable antioxidants.

There are different types of antioxidants, so here are some of my favorites and where you can find them.

Vitamin C	Apples, oranges, lemons
Lycopene	Tomatoes
Lutein	Kale
Flavonols	Cocoa
Anthocyanin	Blueberries, blackberries, raspberries
Quercetin	Apples, onions

Sulforaphane	Broccoli
Catechins	Green tea
Oleocanthal	Extra-virgin olive oil
Curcumin	Turmeric

Effectively, when you eat foods that contain the right ingredients needed to support your health, your body will do exactly that: *support your health.*

Here's my pro tip: Eat more plants. Plants are our friends. Plants have vitamins to support us. You do not have to become a vegetarian or a vegan to have a healthy, symptomless life. That's a myth I will explore in the next chapter. But eating more plants is the best way to get more omega-3s and plant-based antioxidants into your diet, and these ingredients will help you lower your inflammation.

If you can't get enough antioxidants and anti-inflammatories through consumption, you can supplement with:

→ Zinc

→ Turmeric

→ NAC supplement

→ N-acetyl cysteine

Beyond reducing and adding the aforementioned substances to your diet, one of the best ways to fight inflammation is to get tested for it. That's right, I'm about to recommend getting your labs done for the millionth time!

When looking at inflammation, you can focus on underlying gut tests like a GI-MAP. This will help you and your provider identify some underlying issues contributing to unwanted symptoms.

Even if you don't think you have gut problems, you want to pay attention to gut health. Sometimes, gut issues are difficult to pinpoint because the signs and symptoms can happen all over our body. I've had countless women tell me they don't have digestion issues only to find out there is a lot going on behind the scenes that they never quite considered.

Working on gut health is working on the root of your problem. One of the best active steps you can take is to work with a professional to get you on the right gut supplement routine, which should include some probiotics, digestive enzymes, and gut lining repair supplements like L-glutamine. Before we move on, however, I want to dive deeper into two issues I see most commonly and that cause the most pain: weight gain and infertility.

Weight Gain

One of the most common stories I hear concerning PCOS is rapid weight gain. Women find themselves gaining twenty to thirty pounds out of nowhere, feel like a total alien in their own bodies, and then experience extreme depression and anxiety.

I've been there myself, and it's awful.

While weight loss is complicated and highly individualized, I can't write this chapter without directly calling out how hard it is for PCOS ladies to lose weight. We have fundamental hormonal imbalances that make it harder for us to lose weight. Plain and simple. And that's true no matter what hormonal imbalance you are dealing with. Whether it's the insulin piece, the cortisol piece, high testosterone, or anything else, because of how wide the root source of this imbalance can be, we can't approach weight loss by only eating less and moving more like everyone else. We need to be working on hormone balance to achieve lasting, sustainable weight loss.

That's right, we must do twice as much work to lose the weight. And that's okay.

To begin your weight loss journey, you must first start to balance your hormones. Get your labs and review what is off, and then supplement your diet to steady whatever particular imbalance you are facing.

Then, home in on the macronutrient composition of your diet. That means look at your plate to see how many carbs, protein, fat, and fiber you are eating—and make sure that it's right for you. Working with a dietitian can help with this (we do all those calculations for you!), but you also need to pay attention to calories because, while they're not the only important issue, they do matter.

In my own weight loss journey, for years, I totally underestimated how many calories I ate. And for years, this derailed my goals. Once I started getting real with myself about my portions and my macros, I realized how much they matter. If you are struggling to lose weight or have hit a wall, this may be why you're not seeing improvement on the scale even when you're focusing on "eating clean."

If you struggle with your weight, one of the best tips I can give you is to explore and understand what your day looks like when you are eating in a deficit (fewer calories than your body burns) versus what a day looks like when you are overeating (more calories in than your body uses). You can do this by tracking your intake.

Be mindful of what you consume in your breakfast, lunch, and dinner because it adds up quickly. (FYI, working with a dietitian can help you learn how many calories you should consume.)

After all, basic science says this: You will lose weight if you eat *less* than your body is burning. You will gain weight if you eat *more* than your body is burning. That's how basic physiology works. Now, again, macronutrients matter, and your hormones are paramount when we're talking about PCOS weight loss, but pretending calories don't matter in the slightest isn't doing your weight loss journey any favors. To be real, it doesn't matter if you eat the healthiest foods in the world. If you're overeating wild salmon, avocado, or cashews, you will gain weight.

If you want to lose weight and have really been struggling, I urge you to consider calories in and out at some point in your journey. I understand that some people are triggered by counting calories because of a troubled relationship with food, and I respect that. But it can be super helpful to track your caloric intake for just a couple of weeks. I never ask women to track calories and macros forever and ever. But if you track for even two weeks, you will be able to gather so much data about your diet and pinpoint areas of opportunity to help you reach your goals faster!

A basic step you can take if you want to lose weight is cooking more at home in your kitchen. Why? If you want to be in a calorie deficit, it's tough to do if you're always eating out. As someone who used to work in kitchens, I know how much salt, sugar, and fat cooks add to recipes. In those back rooms, people prepare your food with flavor—not health—in mind. Trust me when I say they do not care about your PCOS, hormones, or insulin levels. You don't have to cook up a storm every day. You can just eat simple ingredients that support your health.

Also focus on increasing protein and healthy fats while decreasing empty carbs. Shifting away from carbs allows you to stay away from foods that spike your blood sugar and focus on keeping your glucose steady. That—along with calorie and macro counting—will help you lose unwanted weight.

Infertility

Infertility can be one of the most painful experiences a woman can go through. It can make her question her femininity, her body, her role in society, and her future.

PCOS is the leading cause of infertility globally, so we suffer the psychological toll of not knowing if we will ever be mothers. While not exactly a "root cause" itself, infertility is such an important piece of the PCOS story that I had to bring it up as our final unwanted issue to examine.

If you are under thirty-five, infertility means you haven't gotten pregnant after one year of trying naturally. If this is you, the first step toward battling infertility is an analysis of recent lab data. When I aim to help a woman regulate her period or conceive, I want to know the following: Are her androgens high? Is her estrogen low? Did she just get off birth control? If you are struggling with these issues, I highly recommend you get your labs done annually (or, ideally, every six months).

The Solution

Once we have the data to fix infertility issues, we want to focus all our efforts on getting ovulation and your hormones back on track. That means exercising, eating a diet that supports egg quality, and balancing all the other hormones we reviewed in this chapter. The female period, ovulation, and thus infertility are deeply tied to your hormone levels. If they are out of whack, your body will also tiptoe out of balance.

While I know it's frustrating to hear a broad approach on such a sensitive topic, the truth is infertility is a deeply individual battle. You need specific, expert advice that is aimed at your body. However, my top recommendations for regulating your period, ensuring consistent ovulation, and supporting fertility are as follows:

1. Eat more healthy fats, because cholesterol levels contribute to the creation of thyroid hormones. A recent study by the *American Journal of Clinical Nutrition* found that a steady consumption of healthy fats (olive oil, avocado, fatty fish) can also increase progesterone levels and support healthy ovulation.

2. If you want to punch me after this one, it's okay, but it also might indicate that you really need to focus on this: your stress. Cortisol levels can throw your hormones out of balance. What stresses you is unique to you, as is what calms you. The best piece of advice I can give is to focus on identifying that data and then try to consistently implement a small shift away from the things that stress you and toward a more balanced approach to problem-solving.

3. Moderate your sugar intake. As we've learned by now, all hormones balance each other, and high sugar can throw off your insulin levels, which can lower your progesterone levels. But don't take this to mean "cut out sugar indefinitely." It's all about balance!

4. While we will dive into this shortly, supplements can play a vital role in stabilizing your period hormones. One I often recommend is zinc (it supports your FSH), which supports ovulation, which will—*ding ding ding*—support your progesterone production. Foods rich in zinc are oysters, beef, egg yolks, nuts, and even your grandma's favorite, liver! Others I recommend are magnesium and vitamin C.

Finally, we want to start utilizing the power of data on your fertility journey.

When it comes to your period, pretend like you are a mad scientist, get a secret journal, invent some codes if you must, and start tracking that sh*t.

But don't pull out your phone. I hate to be the bearer of bad news, but tracking your cycle with an app is not accurate. A 2018 study found the accuracy of menstrual cycle app predictions was no better than 21 percent. Yikes!

When I say track your cycle, I mean outside of those predictive apps. Again, I love BBT tracking, which is a tool that measures your body temperature to infer where you are in your cycle. Also, as a bonus, if you are super incompatible with birth control (like me!), tracking a period through a BBT monitor is a great method to prevent pregnancy naturally, without the use of synthetic hormones. Finally, you'll know exactly when to expect Aunt Flo, so no more surprise sneak attack bleeds when you board a plane on your long-awaited vacay.

Here's how to use a BBT tracker. Unlike those annoying BBT thermometers that force you to wake up at the same time every morning, use a wearable BBT tracker like Tempdrop. Put on your bracelet before going to sleep, take it off when you wake up, and check your recorded temp. Nobody has time to reach for that thermometer first

thing in the morning, am I right? And don't let the look of it confuse you. Here's how you read the chart:

→ When your cycle starts, your temperatures will be at their lowest (check out the left side of the chart). Then estrogen will start to climb, but temps will stay low, because estrogen keeps our basal body temps lower.

→ Once you ovulate, progesterone production increases, and you'll see an increase in temperatures as a result (right side).

→ After ovulation, temperatures should remain high until your period, when they start to drop off (or you will see a confirmed pregnancy!).

Your BBT tracker is such a great tool to take control of your health to either prepare for pregnancy, prevent pregnancy, or just understand your unique menstrual cycle (especially for my PCOS gals).

When you do track your cycle accurately, you'll know when you're ovulating. Then getting pregnant becomes much easier (and happens more quickly, too). Plus, when you know which stage of your cycle you're in, you'll finally understand your mood swings, wacky digestion, ever-changing energy levels, and sex drive (hellooooo, body literacy, my queen).

SUPPLEMENTS

As you've probably noticed, supplements are interwoven in my practice as a way to get my clients access to the nutrients they need to thrive. But as compelling as the promise of health in a pill is, you do not need to buy the entire supplement selection at Trader Joe's to be a "health girlie." No, what you really need is a high-quality and intentional selection that supports your exact health needs.

Because PCOS and its symptoms show up differently in every person, it's hard to recommend a specific supplement regimen without knowing information like your medical and health history, your list of allergies or sensitivities, your goals, and what you are currently taking. (Any good dietitian would need to have access to your labs to give you an accurate recommendation for supplement usage.)

Of course, I can make general recommendations like "magnesium can be helpful for sleep and digestion" or "vitamin B_6 can help support healthy progesterone levels," but whether these supplements are the right ones for you is something I need much more information on in order to assess.

Because supplements are so expensive, I highly recommend getting your labs done first and working with a dietitian on your regimen so you don't go wasting dollars on things you don't need. Once you have your labs done, here are some core questions I want my clients to ask themselves as they consider what's right for them:

→ Am I trying to conceive? (If you're thinking about starting your family, a prenatal is highly recommended!)

→ How is my digestion?

→ Am I insulin resistant?

→ What are my stress levels like? (If they are super high, focusing on adrenal health supplements may be a crucial piece of the puzzle.)

If you can't access a dietitian, the answers to these questions are a great place to begin your supplement journey. Once you've answered them, you can start to really think about what gaps in your nutritional and hormonal needs you want to fill.

While there is no one-size-fits-all solution for PCOS ladies, some of my favorite supplements for combating symptoms and alleviating the root cause of your issues are as follows:

→ **Inositol:** Inositol may help support healthy blood sugar balance and lower androgens. Bonus for those who are trying to conceive: It may help boost egg quality!

→ **Vitex:** Vitex may help with healthy ovulation and regulating your cycle. Please don't take this if you have chronically high luteinizing hormone levels (if your ovulation prediction kit is always positive).

→ **Saw Palmetto and Zinc:** These beauties help lower androgens (our male sex hormones that cause so many yucky side effects).

→ **Vitamin D:** Research estimates approximately 67 to 85 percent of women with PCOS are deficient in vitamin D. Getting adequate levels of vitamin D can help your anxiety, depression, ovulation, and sense of overwhelm.

→ **Magnesium:** Magnesium is a supplement, and most Americans are deficient in it. It is beneficial for digestion, mood, and sleep. It calms your nervous system and prevents excess excretion of cortisol. It also assists in blood sugar balance (by helping control insulin production) and may help curb sugar cravings. Finally, it supports your digestion, prevents constipation, and aids in the production of thyroid hormones.

→ **Omega-3 Fatty Acids:** Women with PCOS tend to have higher levels of in-

flammatory markers. Omega-3 fatty acids are a powerful anti-inflammatory! Be careful what you take, though, as not all omega-3s are created equal. Many companies tout their omega-3s as having "2,000 mg omega-3 fish oil," but when you look at the label, they contain only 50 mg of eicosapentaenoic acid (EPA) and 67 mg of docosahexaenoic acid (DHA). It's EPA and DHA that are actually the anti-inflammatory superstars inside "anti-inflammatory supplements," so this is what we're really after! I recommend at least 500 mg of EPA and DHA in an omega-3 supplement.

→ **A Multivitamin:** This can help fill in those nutritional gaps and prevent nutritional deficiencies to keep our metabolism healthy and ready to take on anything that attacks our body.

→ **CoQ10:** It is a powerful antioxidant and my top supplement for the health of your eggs.

→ **Melatonin:** Melatonin is well known for its sleep-inducing effects, but did you know it's also an ovarian antioxidant? Yep, and it helps regulate key sex hormones required for ovulation!

→ **Calcium and B$_6$:** Try 1,200 mg of calcium and 50 mg of vitamin B$_6$ daily. Calcium and B$_6$ have been shown to help with PMS-related feelings of anxiety, sadness, and irritability.

In 2021, after struggling to find adequate supplements, I created VITA-PCOS because I found no affordable supplements on the market for women with PCOS. As a registered dietitian, women's health expert, and PCOS specialist, I knew I had the power to do it, so I did! Here are some of my supplements that can specifically support your PCOS:

→ **Androgen Blocker:** Stops the conversion of certain male hormones (like testosterone) that can lead to hair loss or thinning on your scalp, facial or body hair growth, acne, weight gain or difficulty losing weight, and irregular cycles.

→ **Cortisol Calmer:** Encourages optimal stress levels, calms your mind and body, supports energy levels and mood, and wholly nourishes your adrenals. This will help with anxiety, a high-stress lifestyle, irritability, depression, weight gain (especially around the midsection), difficulty sleeping, fatigue, and mood swings.

→ **Magnesium:** Helps maintain good-quality sleep, healthy bowel movements, and a more stable mood, and it helps reduce PMS.

→ **OvaSupport:** This is an inositol supplement made from vitamin B_8. It works similarly to metformin by balancing your blood sugar and insulin resistance and helps regulate your period, but it's *not* a drug, therefore, no yucky side effects. It also helps with cravings and weight loss and improves egg quality!

Nourishing ourselves with VITA-PCOS is a great first step to managing your symptoms and getting your life back to normal! No matter where you are in your journey, if you don't eat "perfectly" every day (and, like, who does?), supplements can be an excellent way to help fill in the gaps nutrient-wise and bring your symptoms to a manageable level.

MYTH BUSTING

MYTH ONE:
PCOS WOMEN GAIN WEIGHT BECAUSE THEY ARE LAZY.

Hell no. PCOS is a complicated metabolic condition. We have legitimate hormonal imbalances that make losing weight more complicated. PCOS is not a lazy girl condition, but something that one in ten women deal with. While we can—and should—look at calorie counting as a method for sustainable weight loss, we do not gain weight simply because we are lazy.

MYTH TWO:
SELF-CARE IS JUST FOR RICH PEOPLE.

Nope! While there are so many types of self-care, something cheap (like taking a walk while listening to a good podcast) can be just as effective as an expensive facial. What matters is that you get your body out of a chronic stress response and start to move toward homeostasis. Your body doesn't know that the sheet mask from Walgreens cost three dollars, okay? (I won't tell if you won't.)

MYTH THREE:
I NEED EVERY SINGLE SUPPLEMENT EVERY DAY TO BE HEALTHY!

Nah! While it's compelling to buy everything, your wallet and your pantry do not want this. Use your lab data to see what gaps in your hormonal health need to be filled. You must tailor your regimen to your specific needs, not whatever Trader Joe's is selling today. Your body will thank you for this mindfulness!

THE WRAP-UP

This chapter was all about sidestepping PCOS symptoms and addressing the core issues that cause the symptoms. By and large, most symptoms are caused by elevated androgens, low vitamin D, insulin resistance, stress and adrenal dysfunction, and inflammation.

We also touched on two issues so near and dear to the PCOS community: weight gain and infertility. We talked about science-based action plans to lose weight and even to get pregnant, two of the most difficult topics for any woman. I hope you found some clarifying information in this chapter. But know this: No matter what you are trying to overcome—whether it's getting your body back to the place where you feel comfortable and confident, getting rid of facial hair, getting your ovulation back on track, or starting a family—*all those destinations follow a similar path.* And that path is a healthy lifestyle, exercise, and a nourishing, balanced diet.

Getting to the root cause of your PCOS requires you to look at food through the lens of nutrients and see food as the healing entity it really is. The next chapter is going to dive into food myths and nutrition and explore the full narrative of how food can support a fully organic way to take back your power and come to a neutral place for your PCOS.

NITTY-GRITTY NUTRITION

. . . .

The Power of Being Healthy(ish)

Emily can't seem to keep the weight off, even though she's had PCOS, like, forever. When she was younger, she saw her parents lose weight with the Atkins diet, so, in her late twenties, she decided to try it as a last resort. That meant no carbs. No carbs at all. So, when her weight started to creep up in her late twenties, she lost ten pounds by eating only meat and cheese. While her cholesterol shot up, she thought it was fine. Little did she know she would gain and lose that ten pounds for the next decade and that cholesterol would become a problem.

While she was battling her waistline and her cholesterol levels were rising, Emily had a successful venture into digital marketing. When the time was right, she met the right man and had a few kids. Everything was on track for what she imagined for herself . . . everything except this extra freakin' weight she was carrying around her middle. The last time she weighed herself, the ten had ballooned into an astonishing thirty pounds. Gosh. Despite her education and accomplishments, she had no idea how to get the weight off.

It wasn't exactly her fault. Emily grew up on what's called the standard American diet: lots of hamburgers, dairy, butter, and a slice of tomato for color. Her exemplary nurse mom got home late at night and fed her store-bought mac and cheese. Poor Emily didn't get much better nutrients at school. (Did you know that the US government sometimes counts pizza as a vegetable if it has more than half a cup of tomato sauce?)

Emily's education, while robust in very useful topics like trigonometry and geometry, had almost no classes on nutrition. All she remembers was a vague food pyramid thrown at her exactly once in fourth grade.

Now, firmly in her mid-thirties, she was responsible for feeding her own kids. She wanted to do better, but she often came home exhausted, so she put some microwaved chicken nuggets on the table and ate them herself.

Then everything changed. Emily had her annual doctor's appointment, where she got some pretty scary news: Her blood work came back abnormal. She had really high cholesterol, triglycerides, and blood pressure. Her doctor, an older man, looked her up and down. "Didn't you have your kids five years ago? Isn't it time you lost the baby weight? You better start now because you've become prediabetic."

Bright red, Emily rushed out the door into the air-conditioned hallway, and under the fluorescent lighting, it finally hit her. "This weight is seriously impacting my health."

She went home, collapsed on the couch, and went straight to Dr. Google. After a little research, and a lot of over-whelm, the truth became apparent. She had to learn about nutrition or face super scary consequences. Never one to back down from a challenge, Emily found a dietitian (it was me), and we got to work!

With a fierce determination familiar to us mamas, Emily buckled down. She realized it was time for her to get the tools, make the changes, and get this food thing under control. Rather than just give her directions, I focused on educating Emily on what is in our food and how those chemicals affect our health. She needed to get the right nutrients in her body, exercise more, and put fewer calories in to reverse her prediabetes diagnosis.

And girl, she *did*. Emily and I worked diligently on creating a meal plan that was accessible, affordable, and impactful. We learned all about macros, micros, anti-inflammatories, and how to lose weight without hating yourself. We learned that carbs should not be avoided entirely (the human body needs them to function). We also covered why eating well can be so important for balancing hormones and how that balancing act is truly the linchpin for long, steady health and longevity.

And, girl, we definitely covered the fact that she (or anyone, really) didn't need to spend a million hours a week at SoulCycle to be a #healthgirlie. Or only shop at Whole Foods. Or play that vegan game. Or only eat cheese and meat. Or wake up at 4:00 A.M., light a candle, and count your calories from yesterday in a gilded journal sold exclusively at Goop.

Nope. All Emily had to do was learn to eat healthy most of the time. Not all the time. Just most of the time.

Sound good to you? Well, you can do it, too.

• •

It's no secret that many women have a hard time with their weight and, thus, have a complicated relationship with food. A recent study found that "56 percent of women say they are dissatisfied with their overall appearance" and "the overwhelming majority of women—89 percent—want to lose weight." As a dietitian, it makes me *super* upset. Because of all the negative comments women get about their body size, it makes it that much harder for them to achieve a better, sustainable, and healthy relationship with food. And while I'm all in for losing weight for health, before we go into this conversation, we have to talk about body image.

Women have been bombarded their whole lives with unrealistic expectations of beauty, and this has only gotten worse with the proliferation of social media. Now, if we feel that we aren't thin with big butts and boobs, then we are just . . . well . . . a failure. And that isn't good.

Girls! Those expectations (super skinny with double Ds and a juicy butt) were made by men and then executed by a computer (Photoshop and AI). We can't all be Kim Kardashian, nor should we try to be. We also don't have a team of people ready, willing, and able to make us always look our best. We can't compare our bodies to what we see in the media.

With the pressures put on women by society and how much money companies make from women hating themselves, it's hard for women to have a healthy relationship with eating. I see it all the time in my practice: Women have a difficult time learning about health and weight loss without getting into disordered eating habits. What is disordered eating? Well, it's anything that falls into extreme categories, like not eating certain food groups at all (carbs), starving yourself, or even binge eating.

If you do struggle with these patterns and

habits, I highly recommend you talk to a counselor or seek support, because I'm not an expert in this. But I wanted to mention it because I've seen it show up repeatedly as I've counseled women around their diets and helped them get into healthier eating habits.

The last thing I want for any woman is for them to feel so bad about their bodies they starve themselves (and consequently send their hormones on a badly built rocket ship). If they do that, they might lose weight only to gain it all back.

We aren't going to do that here.

What we *want* to do is reestablish your relationship with the word *diet*. For me, the word *diet* is not a demand to reduce consumption but rather a consideration of how you are fueling your body and thus, in many ways, a consideration of how you are fueling your *life*. The food we eat, after all, is the very basis of how our body functions. Without the right vitamins and minerals, our body can't function properly.

Food, in short, is fuel.

Given all the sh*t society throws at us PCOS ladies (we are told that we aren't feminine because of this disorder, that we are lazy, fat, and at fault for our symptoms), we deserve the best d*mn fuel there is! But, babes, eating well is not just about losing weight. It's about learning to love yourself in a new language. We want to eat healthy be-cause we deserve all the benefits and well-ness that come with it.

We want to eat healthy because we love ourselves.

Look at yourself in the mirror, hips and thighs and all of it, and say, "I love you. I deserve to be healthy. I am worthy of a long, lovely life. I love my body enough to learn about food. I love you enough to make life-style changes. I will love this body to help you avoid chronic illness. And I love you enough to have that spicy margarita every once in a while."

When you learn to love yourself, you can see the truth: that you are wonderful and in complete control of your body, health, and mindset. With that in your back pocket, you can learn to act on and implement the changes you want for your health and weight. Even with PCOS, you can shed pounds and feel good in those jeans!

Hopefully, with the tools, tricks, and knowledge I've outlined in this chapter, eating well will not be difficult or expensive. It might be easy, affordable, and desirable.

And yes, eating well can be affordable. Not cheap but affordable. While we all might want to chalk up our diet to dollars, it's not an equal exchange. Eating well is an investment in our future self: What we eat now will directly affect our health down the line. While health food stores want you to think how much you spend equals how healthy you are, that's just not the case. You can use affordable, simple, fresh ingredients and still go miles on your health reboot journey. How? That's why I wrote this chapter.

This part of the book is all about learning to eat on a budget, how anyone can use their grocery list to conquer their hormones and waistlines, and how food is a tool to extend our lives!

EATING HEALTHY . . . CAN BE FUN (YEAH! I SAID IT!)

When I say brussels sprouts, you might think of a soggy, stinky side dish your mom may have shoved on your plate as a kid. You probably thought your mom was just trying to make you eat some healthy sh*t, and when it tasted terrible, you decided you unequivocally hated healthy foods. Given that experience, I'm willing to bet you still don't associate healthy eating with the joy of food. Who wants to eat a brussels sprout when they could grab a pizza?

It turns out that trade-off (carb to veggie) is hardwired into human biology. We want carbs because, back in our caveman days, they were harder to come by, so we valued them more. We also just want carbs because they are delicious, point blank. The truth is, even if you are on a weight loss journey, you can still have that carb. But if you are also interested in moving the needle on your health journey and losing a few pounds, there are a few things you can add

to your carbs that will help you lose weight and steady your blood sugar: protein and fiber.

Protein is so useful for your body and doesn't have to come in the form of red meat. No, it can be legumes, dairy, nuts, seeds, tofu, poultry, and fish, too.

Fiber is found in what dietitians call complex carbohydrates and in fruits, veggies, grains, and legumes.

Both substances are critical to feeling full and achieving weight loss goals. Both are also magical for helping control blood sugar. Here's what I'm talking about: If you eat a bowl of mac and cheese, your blood sugar will not be happy. But if you add a li'l broccoli and some roasted chicken to that same mac and cheese, those ingredients will help counteract the spike in glucose that the pasta will cause, and the protein and fiber make you feel full for longer, and keep your insulin levels steady eddie. And that's what you want: steady blood sugar. Healthy blood sugar will help anyone reverse a prediabetic condition, fight a type 2 diabetes diagnosis, and lose any unwanted weight.

Getting steady blood sugar levels (and getting healthy) is all about making small changes. You don't have to give up your favorite childhood foods to get healthy. Nope. What you do have to change is your mindset about eating and be sure to incorporate lots of protein and fiber.

Black-and-White Thinking

I see black-and-white thinking when it comes to food all the time. Here's what I'm talking about: How many Mondays have you proclaimed you would start your diet and commit to going to the gym only to give up by Friday because you want to go out with your friends to get Italian food? Then Saturday comes, and you've already shot it to hell with some creamy Alfredo sauce, so you just decide that you'll start again on Monday.

The week goes great until Friday comes, and you drink a whole bottle of wine with your friends, and you give up again, ada-

mantly yelling to anyone who'll listen that you will start your diet again on Monday.

Three months later, you're seven pounds heavier and you kind of hate yourself.

This black-and-white/all-or-nothing cycle was mine for a while, and it drove me nuts. I got nowhere fast and ended up heavier than I had ever been. I've seen hundreds of women go through the toxic cycle of all in or all out on their wellness, only to find the all out is leading them toward a prediabetes condition, heightened unwanted PCOS symptoms, or other chronic illnesses.

The hard truth is that when it comes to your health, there are no good or bad days. Even if you have a scone in the morning, it doesn't mean that you can't eat well for the rest of the day. The same goes for food: There are no good or bad foods. All foods can fit into a healthy, balanced lifestyle. It's just figuring out how much and when. That's why I don't preach all-or-nothing diets. We must learn to eat for our future selves while not making our current selves miserable!

And that art is all about #balance. To achieve that balance, though, we have to start with some nutrient basics!

THE FOUR NUTRIENTS

Babe, welcome to the nutrition class you never got in school. While I could go on and on about how awful it is that Americans basically never learn about nutrition (and doctors only get one class), we're about to turn that ship around.

In this Nutrition 101 review, we are going to start with covering the four kinds of nutrients that our body needs. Not "needs" like we need our Amazon Prime account, but what our body actually requires on a biological basis. Here's what they are:

1. Macronutrients: These include carbs, protein, fat, and I like to also tack on fiber.

2. Micronutrients: This is a fancy word for vitamins and minerals.

3. Antioxidants: These help our body fight off free radicals that cause cancer.

4. Anti-inflammatories: These are specific foods containing anti-inflammatory ingredients.

Without adequate amounts of all four of these nutrients, our body has no chance to be healthy. And yes, that includes carbs.

THE TABOO MACROS: CARBS

Despite the negative connotations that carbs have, they fall under the category of macros, and our bodies need them to function! So, let's bust this myth right here: While many doctors tell PCOS patients to cut carbs to lose weight (and yes, cutting carbs to a degree can be helpful to manage weight and keep insulin healthy), we can't cut carbs forever for so many reasons. Who wants to live life without a bagel ever again? Def not me!

We can't completely cut out carbs because they are not just found in bread, starches, and rice. Fruit and vegetables also have carbs. Did you know a banana has 22.8 g of carbs and is a healthy source of fiber, vitamins B_6 and C, and potassium?

The trick with carbs is to pick the complex ones, like bananas, that will digest slowly and have a multitude of other nutrients, antioxidants, and other benefits. Things like barley, farro, quinoa, and whole-wheat bread are carbs but are better for your blood sugar than white bread, white rice, and other ultraprocessed foods.

We want to pick complex carbs because they digest slower in our system and don't spike our blood sugar as dramatically. Again, spiking blood sugar is something that all people—not just PCOS warriors—should aim to avoid because it is the precursor to chronic lifestyle diseases.

THE TABOO TWIN: FATS

Fats are our friends *and* food. (Does anyone get the *Finding Nemo* reference? Just me? Oh well.) Despite what the media might have you think, eating fats won't make you fat. In fact, fats are the building blocks of our hormones. When I say "fats," I'm referring to the overarching nutrition term for structural fats, body fat, and dietary fats. Structural fats are super important for our body's functioning. They are the chemical building blocks for our cells, hormones, and brain. Body fat is exactly what it sounds like: that extra li'l jiggle on your hips, thighs, and wherever else. A little bit is good for you. Our fat actually protects our organs from impact, which is why it can be evolutionarily harder to lose!

Body fat is also where our body stores extra energy and can help us stay insulated during the colder months. However, body fat is not the same as dietary fats and isn't directly derived from fats we consume.

Health problems can arise when we deprive ourselves of healthy fats and dietary cholesterol. Dietary fats, which can be sourced from animals (milk, steak, fish, etc.) and plants (avocados, nuts, oils), help hold your body together! Women need these nutrients to help stabilize their blood sugar, balance their hormones, and keep their bodily fluids flowing well.

PROTEIN

When I think of protein, I think of my college boyfriend who worked his butt off to get swole. The kid would drink two protein shakes daily, stuff himself with turkey and chicken for lunch, and then pound ground beef for dinner. I remember going over to his apartment after classes and not seeing one vegetable in the fridge.

As a couple, we didn't work out (his poop stank from not eating enough fiber, and so did his attitude), but I did learn a lot about the concept of protein from him. Protein isn't just for the gym bros. Proteins are large molecules that comprise long chains of amino acids and can help our bodies do many different types of work: replicating DNA, providing structure to our cells, and helping our body move molecules from one location to another.

In terms of our diet, consuming protein helps us stabilize our blood sugar and makes our hormones rise and fall more steadily. While everything depends on personal goals, I have found women should aim for 20 to 30 g of protein per meal or 30 to 40 percent of their daily calories. Protein keeps us fuller longer (which helps us cut down on cravings), so up the protein, girls!

While I can't give you the exact amount of protein grams you should eat because we're all unique little snowflakes (and that number depends on lots of factors, including your height, weight, age, and weight goals), make sure you're filling up on enough protein to feel good. For my PCOS ladies, eating a high-protein diet can help us reduce unwanted mood swings, cravings, fatigue, period issues, and PCOS symptoms like facial hair and weight gain.

If that sounds good to you, consider these options for how to get more protein in your diet. If you are eating pasta, try swapping it out for a chickpea version instead! (My favorite, and this is not an ad, is Banza pasta! It's very good.) If you love rice and can't see yourself giving it up, try swapping it out occasionally for quinoa (which has a much higher protein content). And finally, find a protein powder you like, and swoosh it around in anything that can handle it! (I like to put it in my smoothies and oats.)

Pro tip: Get some protein early in the day. And yes, I'm talking about breakfast. When you eat breakfast, especially a low-sugar, high-protein breakfast, you stabilize your blood sugar and give your body the fuel you need to get through the day. Your breakfast doesn't have to be fancy or complex or Insta-worthy. It could look like adding collagen and peanut butter to your oats, a banana and full-fat milk to your cereal, and an egg and avo to your toast. Again, fat, fiber, and protein slow glucose absorption into your bloodstream, so you aren't sent on a blood sugar roller-coaster ride.

FIBER

You've probably heard of fiber from a random Google search if you felt a little blocked up. And yes, if you gotta poo, fiber is great. But it's so much more than just for constipation emergencies.

As a dietitian, I talk about fiber all day errrry day. Like, I'm borderline annoying about it. Fiber is crucial for healthy hormone levels because it helps our body excrete estrogen, keeps our blood sugar balanced better, and keeps us fuller longer in between meals/snacks. But what is fiber? It's an indigestible material found in natural foods, and it helps you go! Here are my five favorite ways to sneak more fiber into your diet:

1. Put chia seeds in your smoothie.

2. Swap regular pasta for bean-based pasta.

3. Add beans to your soup.

4. Don't peel your produce.

5. Add avocado to your salad.

By incorporating more fiber into your diet, you are helping your body smoothly move (pun intended) in the right direction!

Fruit, as much as it's demonized in the health world, is one of our best natural sources of fiber. Whole fresh fruit comes packed with its own natural supply of fiber to negate the rapid absorption of fructose into your bloodstream, meaning you won't go on a blood sugar roller coaster. It is impossible to overeat fructose in fruit because it is full of fiber, water, and body-benefiting phytonutrients. So, the next time you hear someone bashing a banana, tell 'em what's good.

I can't tell you how many patients ask me if they can eat fruit. Truth bomb: Life without any fruit is not a life I would ever want to live and not a life you ever need to live.

In my practice, I consider fruit a carbohydrate. They're full of the primary sugars glucose and fructose but also contain hefty amounts of fiber and antioxidants. Despite all the myths that PCOS ladies should subscribe to a keto or no-carb diet (and I will debunk those myths shortly), for now, all you need to know is that fruit can fit into a healthy PCOS eating routine.

If you want to eat that mango, go right ahead. But, because we do have PCOS, we want to consider the following guidelines to make sure we aren't spiking our blood sugar unnecessarily:

→ **Eat fruit in moderation.** This means scaling back on your normal portion sizes and opting for smaller servings. For example, instead of 1 cup of grapes for a snack, try ⅓ cup.

→ **Pair fruit with a little protein and/or fat.** This will help negate the blood sugar spike that normally accompanies eating fruit on its own. For example, try a hard-boiled egg with half of an apple or nuts with half of a banana.

→ **Maintain a healthy attitude around fruit.** Guess what will happen if you completely avoid eating fruit? Spoiler alert: You will crave it and then binge on it later. Focus on making small, healthy changes slowly rather than going hard-core keto overnight and then fighting your body on it later.

Pro Tip!

If you are a little overwhelmed by all this information, here's something to help you: the skill of food sequencing! Research shows eating your veggies and protein *before* your carbs reduces blood sugar spikes, improves weight loss efforts, and reduces PCOS symptoms. Think asparagus and salmon, then buttered pasta!

Why? Protein and fiber before a carb help reduce post-meal glucose and insulin spikes and allow the body to convert these food sources into sustainable energy slowly. Protein, fat, and fiber delay gastric emptying (the rate at which food exits the stomach), so you'll feel full and satisfied with more energy and fewer cravings afterward.

Boo-ya!

WHAT'S UP, MICRONUTRIENTS?!

Girls, as we know, our body is a powerful beast. It is always operating, even when we're sleeping. And the human body is always trying to move toward balance except, you know, if we have PCOS. Then we have to help it out a little bit. One of the best ways anyone can support their body is by eating enough micronutrients, often referred to as vitamins and minerals. These substances, with the exception of vitamin D, are not produced in the body and must be derived from the diet.

There are literally so many vitamins and minerals the body needs that I'm going to run through them at the end of this chapter! But here are some of the heavy hitters:

Zinc

This teeny, little micronutrient has big health impacts on the female body. It is a powerful anti-inflammatory and hormone regulator and can help relieve period pain and cramping. A little bit can help stimulate ovulation by nourishing your eggs.

Zinc also blocks excess androgens by inhibiting the enzyme 5-alpha-reductase, which is a necessity in treating acne and hirsutism in women with PCOS. And it can help clear skin by opening pores and reducing keratin production. Finally, this powerful little mineral supports the reduction of cortisol (your stress response) for better moods and proper hormone balance.

Your body cannot store zinc, so you must get enough of this mineral through your diet. Vegetarians, vegans, and predominantly plant-based babes listen up! The best sources of zinc are oysters and red meat, so considering a supplement is vital. Many multivitamins and prenatals include zinc, so check the back of your bottle. I prefer zinc picolinate and zinc citrate, as these are highly absorbable by the body. Zinc is also depleted by hormonal birth control, alcohol, and certain meds, so if any of these apply to you, supplement ya zinc.

Vitamin C

Who loves a good old dose of citrus? I know I do! There's nothing more satisfying than a perfect little mandarin, but did you know these citrus fruits have huge doses of vitamin C? And nope, it's not quite the same as the vitamin C packets your mom gave you when you were sick. When it comes to our immune system, vitamin C helps white blood cells function more effectively, strengthens our skin's defense system, and helps wounds heal faster.

Vitamin C is naturally found in a lot of frozen foods (like berries and broccoli, which can help bring down the grocery budget!), bell peppers, guava, and even kiwifruit!

While fresh produce can get expensive, I will tell you a secret: That frozen stuff is just as good. It also doesn't go bad, rot in the bottom of your fridge, and then guilt you for letting it go bad. Nope, the frozen stuff can just sit there so you can use it at your convenience. This is one of the many ways we can keep to our budget and eat healthy. I love a pretty Instagram meal, but I deeply hate cutting up raw broccoli. (Is it me, or do those little bits of broccoli just get everywhere? Ugh!) When I use frozen broccoli, I don't have to worry about that, and my family gets all the nutrients available in the frozen form.

Cheap + easy = I'm way more likely to eat my veggies!

Iron

If you've ever lost a lot of blood, felt weak, or noticed some hair loss, it's possible your iron is low. Before you go HAM on the iron supplements, make sure you're getting your iron absorbed with a hefty dose of vitamin C.

Vitamin C and iron (especially plant-based iron) are basically besties. Plant-based iron (non-heme iron) is not as easily absorbed by the body as, say, something like steak or pork. But vitamin C enhances plant-based iron's absorption by capturing it and storing it in a form that's easier for your body to take in and use. Be sure to pair your iron-rich plant-based foods with something high in vitamin C when you're eating them together. Foods high in plant-based iron are dark leafy green veggies like spinach and kale, beans, fortified cereals, dried fruits, and quinoa.

Omega-3s

If you're not a big fan of fish, that's no excuse to skimp on your omega-3 fatty acids. These nutritional powerhouses reduce levels of inflammation in the body. As we've learned, research demonstrates that women with PCOS are in a chronic state of low-grade inflammation, meaning we have to work extra hard at mitigating inflammatory processes in our bodies. What is the best way to do this naturally? By eating a diet high in anti-inflammatories and incorporating more omega-3 fatty acids into our diet! Omega-3 fatty acids are also important for weight loss efforts. Researchers have suggested that fish oil omega-3s may help people lose weight more easily.

Clinical studies show omega-3s reduce prostaglandins, which are the lipid compounds responsible for period cramps and breast tenderness. I recommend 500 mg of omega-3 fatty acids daily. When we're talking about omega-3s, it's really the EPA and DHA we're after! These two types of omega-3s are readily absorbed and utilized by our bodies to combat inflammation. Often, you will hear that walnuts, flaxseed, chia seeds, and hemp seeds are great sources of omega-3s. While this is true, they only contain alpha-lipoic acid (ALA), a form of omega-3 converted in our bodies at a rate of less than 10 percent. So, while you shouldn't steer away from these foods, it's best to take in omega-3s that have high levels of EPA and DHA.

Overall, read the labels, girls. Not all supplements are created equal.

Magnesium

Magical magnesium! This little mineral does wonders for your body. It is used for 600 cellular reactions, including your brain and heart functioning, to make your muscles contract. It also helps lower your blood sugar. It is the fourth most abundant mineral in your body. Despite how critical this is, up to 68 percent of American adults don't meet the recommended daily intake. Low levels of this critical vitamin can contribute to weakness, depression, high blood pressure, and even heart disease. Taking magnesium can be great for your mood, digestion, and sleep, and it also helps decrease insulin resistance and may serve as a key weight loss aid.

Take it at night to help your muscles relax and help you go to sleep. Take that mag and get some deep zzzs and some good poops.

Making sure you get the right vitamins is critical to your current and long-term health. Feeding your body the right amount of micronutrients will move the body toward balance and make any goals like weight loss more easily achievable. If you don't, your body will feel deprived of the (very) necessary nutrients it needs to survive and won't be optimized at its highest potential. When you get the right vitamins, you are supporting your health and moving your physical condition toward optimal balance.

Rather than deprive yourself of food in efforts to make yourself thin, when you take effort and care to feed your body the right stuff, your body will thank you by getting stronger, healthier, less inflamed, and overall more in alignment with whatever goal you want to achieve, whether that be weight loss, pregnancy, or just reducing unwanted symptoms. You need legitimate micros for your body to thrive.

Antioxidants

Another food group we PCOS ladies (and all humans) need is antioxidants.

Even when we are relaxing, our body—on a cellular level—is doing tons of work. Specifically, our body's trillion cells are constantly (like, literally every second) fighting free radicals. Free radicals are formed from our body's natural system for transforming food into energy. But free radicals can also come from regular exposure to smoke, air pollution, and even sunlight! Excessive exposure to free radicals can increase our chances of cancer, can damage our cells, and can even lead to chronic diseases.

One of our body's best natural defenses for free radicals is something found naturally in foods: antioxidants. Antioxidants work by giving their energy to cells; that energy helps our cells stay healthy and make repairs. Antioxidants are also involved in mechanisms that repair DNA and maintain the health of cells.

The best news is that foods high in antioxidants are also commonly frozen, such as berries, spinach, broccoli, and cauliflower. Studies show that high consumption of these foods is better for your overall health and can even prevent visible signs of aging.

Women with PCOS want to be extra intentional about their antioxidant consumption because we have more free radicals and inflammation than other folks (I know, great news, right?). Because we have unstable hormones, we are at an increased risk for all the negative effects free radicals—

and overall inflammation—can cause. A recent study found that when PCOS women used antioxidant supplements, they experienced improved insulin sensitivity and better reactions to health-threatening conditions like obesity and androgen excess.

While, as a dietitian, I do advocate for you to get most of your nutrients, micronutrients, antioxidants, and anti-inflammatories through your diet, the right supplements are always a good alternative if it's unlikely you'll get what you need through food (and girl, we all don't eat right 100 percent of the time. Even I take supplements when it matters most!).

If you want a complete list of what foods have, check out this chart:

NUTRIENT	BENEFIT	FOODS
Vitamin C	Vitamin C is like that gentle nurse with the kind smile getting you patched up. This vitamin is an antioxidant that helps your body heal its wounds and maintain healthy tissue. It's also important for strong teeth and gums, progesterone levels and ovulation, and absorbing iron.	Broccoli Brussels sprouts Cabbage Cauliflower Citrus fruits Potatoes Spinach Strawberries Tomatoes Tomato juice
Vitamin B_{12}	Vitamin B_{12} is the electrician checking up on the house. It's important for getting the house powered up (metabolism—converting food into energy) and making sure all the wiring in your nervous system is working. It also helps with energy levels, helps form red blood cells, and prevents hair loss.	Dairy products Eggs Liver Nutritional yeast Red meat Seafood

NUTRIENT	BENEFIT	FOODS
Vitamin E	Vitamin E is that gorgeous model whose skin is always perfection. If you're getting the right amount of vitamin E, your skin will stay healthy and vibrant! This antioxidant helps form red blood cells, assists with vitamin K usage in the body, and also goes by tocopherol.	Kiwifruit Mangos Nuts Seeds Tomatoes Vegetable oils
Vitamin D	Everybody's met vitamin D before. It's like I don't even have to introduce her. She shows up in your body after being in the sun. With 10 to 15 minutes of sunlight three times a week, the vitamin D made by your body will help you better absorb calcium, which you need for strong teeth and bones. Remember, women with PCOS are chronically deficient in vitamin D and need it to keep periods regular.	Egg yolks Fatty fish like salmon Some mushrooms
Vitamin B_6	Vitamin B_6 is a meat lover! It's a vitamin that lets the proteins in your body do their jobs in making all the necessary chemical reactions happen. But the more protein you eat, the more vitamin B_6 your body will need. It also helps form red blood cells, maintains brain function, and also goes by pyridoxine.	Bananas Oats Peanuts Pork Poultry Some fish Soybeans Wheat germ
Vitamin B_9	Vitamin B_9 is also known as folate and can be found added in foods in the form of folic acid. It's vitamin B_{12}'s best friend, and these two work together to help form red blood cells. It's also something you want to make sure you're getting enough of if you're pregnant because it's used in DNA production, and low levels of folate can cause birth defects like spina bifida.	Asparagus Broccoli Beans Brussels sprouts Dark green leafy vegetables, including romaine lettuce, spinach, turnip greens Fresh fruits Fruit juices Liver Peanuts Sunflower seeds Whole grains
Iron	I never really thought about how our bodies need metals in them, but iron is necessary for our growth, development, and hormones. It's used to make proteins that move oxygen from our cells to all parts of our bodies, and it prevents fatigue and hair loss.	Heme sources, including red meat, seafood Non-heme sources, including spinach, iron-fortified breads and cereals, broccoli, beans (The body does not absorb non-heme sources as effectively.)

NUTRIENT	BENEFIT	FOODS
Vitamin K	Vitamin K holds back the floodgates when your blood is trying to escape (Hint: The blood is supposed to stay in your body). It's needed for blood clotting to stop bleeding at injured vessels, and studies suggest it also strengthens your bones.	Broccoli Brussels sprouts Cabbage Green leafy vegetables, including collard and turnip greens, kale, spinach Lettuces
Vitamin B$_7$	B$_7$ or biotin is the freestyle dancer of our vitamins because it loves to break it down. It helps break down and metabolize proteins, carbohydrates, and fats. It also helps make hormones and cholesterol. Biotin can be taken as a supplement for hair growth.	Avocados Beef liver Eggs (cooked) Nuts Pork Salmon Seeds Sweet potatoes
Choline	Choline is our brainiac nerd. It's important for the development of our brains during pregnancy; after that, it helps the brain operate and communicate with the rest of the body. Low choline may make your liver swell.	Beef Broccoli Cauliflower Chicken breast Dairy Egg yolks Fish Soy
Selenium	We need this mineral for our metabolism, immune system, and thyroid.	Brazil nuts Organ meats Seafood
Potassium	Potassium is our one-woman band. The list can go on and on, but here are a few duties of potassium: lowers blood pressure; helps send nerve signals; regulates fluids and muscle contractions; reduces water retention; and protects against stroke, osteoporosis, and kidney stones.	Apricots Bananas Bell peppers Black beans Cantaloupe Dates Honeydew Oranges Prunes Raisins

NUTRIENT	BENEFIT	FOODS
Sodium	Considering the American diet, I'm willing to bet you're already getting plenty of salt and sodium, but I'll still let you in on why we need sodium in our bodies: It keeps fluids in balance and helps with nerve and muscle function.	Beans with salt added Broth with salt added Salted nuts Smoked, cured, salted or canned meat, fish, or poultry including anchovies, bacon, caviar, cold cuts, frankfurters, ham, sardines, sausage Table salt
Zinc	Another one-man band (maybe potassium and zinc should just start a band together). Zinc is found in plant foods, animal foods, and supplements and can boost immune function, help make DNA and cells, keep skin healthy, protect against inflammation and acne, and for women with PCOS, zinc can help with facial hair issues.	Beef Cashews and other nuts Chickpeas and other legumes Crab Lobster Oats Oysters Pork
Copper	We don't talk about copper as much as iron, but it's still important for making red blood cells and strengthening your immune system. It also keeps nerve cells healthy, helps make energy, helps absorb iron, acts as an antioxidant, and helps form collagen for bones and connective tissue.	Beans Black pepper Cocoa Dark leafy greens Dried fruits such as prunes Nuts Organ meats like kidneys and liver Oysters and other shellfish Potatoes Whole grains Yeast
Calcium	We can't forget one of our star performers: the strongman, calcium. Calcium makes our bones and teeth strong, protecting us against osteoporosis.	Almonds Blackstrap molasses Brazil nuts Dairy products, including buttermilk, cheeses, yogurt Dried beans Green leafy vegetables, including bok choy, broccoli, Chinese cabbage, collards, kale, mustard greens, turnip greens Salmon and sardines canned with their soft bones Sunflower seeds Tahini

NUTRIENT	BENEFIT	FOODS
Magnesium	Magnesium is our comfy homebody who's all about self-care and relaxing bubble baths. This nutrient is amazing for keeping your mood up, keeping your heartbeat nice and steady, and helping with all that resting and digesting. It also maintains normal nerve and muscle function, supports immune function, and stabilizes glucose levels.	Almonds Avocados Black beans Cashews Dark chocolate Edamame Peanuts Quinoa Spinach Whole wheat
Iodine	Iodine is all about the hormones, baby. It's key for making thyroid hormones specifically, which control metabolism and help with bone and brain development.	Beef liver Chicken Dairy, including cheese, milk, yogurt Eggs Fish and shellfish, including canned tuna, cod, oysters, shrimp Seaweed, including kelp, kombu, nori, wakame Table salts labeled "iodized"
Phosphorus	Don't let calcium take the spotlight when phosphorus is close behind it in helping form bones and teeth. It also helps transfer and store energy from carbohydrates and fats, makes proteins, and makes and repairs cells and tissues.	Dairy Legumes Nuts Poultry Red meat Seafood
Allium	Allium is a brave defender and guardian, shielding us from attacks on all sides. It protects us from cancer, heart disease, inflammation, obesity, diabetes, and harmful microbes while boosting our immune system and neuroprotective capabilities.	Chives Garlic Leeks Onions Scallions
Anthocyanins	You don't have to know how to pronounce it, but anthocyanins are another brave defender, protecting us against high blood pressure, heart disease, neurological disease, and cancer.	Berries Currants Grains Grapes Red to purplish and purplish to blue-colored leafy vegetables Roots Some tropical fruits Tubers

NUTRIENT	BENEFIT	FOODS
Carotenoids	Carotenoids are a whole family of antioxidants that protect you from free radicals. Check out the family of fruits and veggies that have these antioxidants (the egg yolks are welcome to the family reunion, too).	Avocados Bell peppers Cantaloupe Carrots Corn Egg yolks Kale Mangos Oranges Pumpkin Spinach Summer squash Tomatoes Watermelon Yams Yellow-fleshed fruits
Capsaicin	This is what makes chile peppers feel like they're catching your mouth on fire! Despite the burn, capsaicin can actually reduce inflammation and help your heart. Studies suggest that it can slightly increase metabolism and decrease appetite.	Bell peppers Cayenne peppers Jalapeño peppers Other chile peppers
Tannins/ Catechins	Tannins and catechins can have an intense bitter taste but have great antioxidant and anti-inflammatory effects.	Apricots Black grapes Broad beans Cacao Cereals Coffee Legume seeds Nuts Peas Some leafy green vegetables Strawberries Tea Wine
Isoflavones	The misunderstood one . . . isoflavones. The isoflavones in soy (and legume seeds) can be given a bad name, but in moderation, they can actually protect you from heart disease, hormonal cancers, osteoporosis, and cognitive decline.	Legume seeds, including beans, lentils, peas Soy and its products

NUTRIENT	BENEFIT	FOODS
Lignans	You don't have to know all the fancy words that go with understanding what lignans do; just know that they can help you fight cancer and act as antioxidants.	Barley Buckwheat Flax Legumes Millet Nuts Oats Rye Sesame seeds Wheat
Phytic Acid	Even though phytic acid is considered an anti-nutrient, as long as your diet is balanced, phytic acids will serve as great antioxidants. They may also help prevent cancer and osteoporosis.	Grains, including oats, rice, whole wheat Legumes, including black beans, kidney beans, lentils, peanuts, pinto beans, soybeans Nuts and seeds, including almonds, pine nuts, sesame seeds, walnuts
Saponins	Another (natural) chemical that can leave a bitter taste on your tongue. Saponins are great antioxidants that reduce free radicals and oxidative stress.	Asparagus Garlic Ginseng Legumes, including broad beans, kidney beans, lentils Licorice Oats Onions Spinach Sugar beets Tea Yams
Limonoids	Add limonoids to our growing army of defenders. They give us protection from cancer, bacteria, fungus, malaria, and viruses.	Bergamots Grapefruits Lemons Limes Mandarins Oranges Pomelos

NUTRIENT	BENEFIT	FOODS
Lycopene	Lycopene is all dressed in red! It gives a reddish hue to the food it's in and boosts your immune system. It also stops oxidation of DNA, lipids, and protein and stops cancer cell growth.	Apricots Cranberries Grapes Melons Papayas Peaches Tomatoes Watermelon
Polyphenols	Polyphenols are the bigger family that isoflavones and lignans come from. Polyphenols protect you from cancer through their antioxidant and anti-inflammatory properties and may even help you fight off infection and disease.	Apples Black currants Black olives Black tea Blueberries Cherries Coffee Dark chocolate Hazelnuts Pecans Plums Strawberries
Sterols	Looking to lower cholesterol? Get more sterols in your diet. Sterols are a stepping stone to making steroid hormones but also help with cell signaling, gene reading, and transport between cells.	Almond butter Cocoa butter oil Macadamia nuts Mayonnaise Olive oil Oregano Paprika Pistachios Sage Sesame oil Sesame seeds Thyme Wheat germ oil
Terpenes	Terpenes are what make lavender and rosemary smell sooo amazing. Once you're done smelling them, you can eat some foods containing terpenes for some anti-inflammatory, antioxidant, antiviral, antidiabetic, and anticancer action.	Apples Citrus fruits Herbs Mangos Spices

NUTRIENT	BENEFIT	FOODS
Zeaxanthin	If you're curious about this one, it's pronounced zee-uh-zan-thn. It's believed to protect our eyes from sun damage.	Corn Eggs Goji berries Grapes Mangos Orange peppers Oranges
Carbo-hydrates	We've got quite the love-hate relationship going on with carbohydrates after all we've learned about them. But we can't live without them. Carbohydrates are a key energy source that helps with glucose levels, insulin metabolism, fermentation for digestion, and other types of metabolism.	Beans Bread Cookies Corn Fruit Fruit juice Lentils Pasta Pastries Peas Potatoes Sweet potatoes Tortillas Winter squash
Fat	"Not all fats." We don't want too much of this around, but we still need the good ones in our lives. The good fats are important for storing energy and supporting our cells. Fats also make hormones, protect organs, keep you warm, and help absorb nutrients.	Avocados Butter Cheese Coconut Fatty red meats Nut/seed butters Nuts Oil Olives Seeds
Protein	So we learned that protein isn't just for the gym bros. We all need it for building tissue all over our bodies. It also repairs tissue, drives metabolic reactions, moves and stores nutrients, keeps pH levels and fluids balanced, and strengthens immune function.	Beans Collagen peptides Cottage cheese Edamame Fish Greek yogurt Lentils Poultry Protein powder Red meat Shellfish Tempeh Tofu

NUTRIENT	BENEFIT	FOODS
Fiber	Fiber! Fiber! Fiber! . . . Tired of hearing about fiber yet? To review, it keeps us fuller longer, which helps us lose weight, and it keeps our blood sugar stable. It also moves waste through our bodies, stops constipation, and keeps our gut microbiota healthy.	Avocados Beans Fruits Lentils Nuts Seeds like chia and flax Vegetables Whole grains

FOODS TO LIMIT

So, we've talked a lot about which foods are best to consume regarding health and are especially good if you have PCOS. If you are interested in shedding some weight, all of these foods will 100 percent support your weight loss goals. But don't get too stuck in "doing the right thing all the time." The trick, with life and in business, is to be all about balance. We want to make sure we are eating our macros, micros, and antioxidants without being too strict about what we can't eat (in other words, foods we might want to reduce that we just love). I say reduce because we don't want to cut out "bad" foods entirely! When we do that, we are more likely to binge our cheat foods when our cravings *hiiit*. All foods—even nachos and margaritas—can be celebrated in moderation, but you have to know what you might want to limit.

Some of the following foods may feel like total duhs to you, but think about how often these foods creep into our diets when we're out and about, at a friend's house, eating at restaurants, or getting takeout/delivery (especially for those of us living in the United States). When we can recognize how much these foods show up, we can be more intentional about our consumption of them.

Sugar

Sugar is really one of the most obvious but difficult foods to cut back on. From juice drinks that masquerade as "health beverages" to tomato and BBQ sauces to granola to flavored yogurt to nut butter to certain protein powders, sugar hides in *everything*! Take a look at the nutrition label on the next page and get familiar with where "sugar" is located:

Nutrition Facts

Serving Size: 6 ounces
Serving Per Container: 1

Amount per serving:

Calories 160	Calories from Fat 25

	% Daily Value
Total Fat 2.5g	4%
Saturated Fat 1.5g	8%
Trans Fat 0g	3%
Cholesterol 10mg	3%
Sodium 105mg	4%
Total Carbohydrate 26g	
Dietary Fiber 0g	
Sugars 25g	
Protein 8g	16%

Vitamin A 0%	**Calcium** 25%
Vitamin C 0%	**Iron** 0%

*Percent Daily Values are based on a 2,000 calorie diet. Your Daily Values may be higher or lower depending on your calorie needs.

Ingredients: Dextrose, fructose, honey, invert sugar, raw sugar, malt syrup, rice syrup, sucrose, xylose, molasses, corn sweetener, fruit juice concentrate, high-fructose, brown sugar, corn syrup, glucose, lactose, maltose, sucrose, evaporated cane juice, agave nectar, cane crystals, cane sugar, crystalline fructose, barley malt, beet sugar, caramel.

Now look at the nutrition label below it. All of these are aliases for added sugar. (Did you know the higher up on a list an ingredient appears, the *more* of it is inside that product? For example, this fake product is made up mostly of dextrose and fructose and has very low amounts of beet sugar and caramel.) I want you to familiarize yourself with this list and become a *nutrition label investigator* the next time you eat something packaged. If possible, try to eat foods with minimal sugar and minimally processed sugar substitutes.

Empty Carbohydrates

When we use the term *empty carb*, what we really mean is *lacking in fiber*. This could be white rice, white bread, white pasta, candy, pastries, cookies, chips, pretzels, bagels, sweetened granolas, and so on. These do nothing but raise our blood sugar, which in turn makes our PCOS worse and throws off our cortisol levels and delicate hormone balance. I know these foods are everywhere (coffee shops, diners, your mama's pantry), so bring healthy, nourishing snacks with you when you head to these places or eat beforehand so that you're not tempted to send your blood sugar for a roller-coaster ride.

Sugar-Sweetened Beverages

These could be sodas (Coke, Pepsi, Fanta, etc.), juice (even if it's "all-natural"), coffee drinks (most Starbucks drinks are loaded with sugar), energy drinks, juice or sparkling juice drinks (like Izze or San Pellegrino), or sports drinks (like Gatorade and vitaminwater). These will skyrocket your blood sugar immediately upon drinking them, causing your PCOS to worsen. And nobody wants that!

SOY

Soy has a bad rap! There are a lot of myths out there about whether soy is good for anyone, specifically for PCOS ladies. And girls, I will come out and say it: We can eat soy, even with PCOS!

How much soy should we eat? As with any food out there, I would never recommend eating something all day, every day! The same goes for soy: I recommend two to three servings a week of whole-food sources of soy, such as:

→ Tofu

→ Tempeh

→ Edamame

→ Soy nuts (You can often find these roasted as yummy, crunchy snacks.)

→ Miso

→ Soy milk (Choose unsweetened plain.)

You might want to limit the ultraprocessed vegan soy hot dogs and burgers! Also, try to pick organic soy when you can. But, babes, stay within these parameters and enjoy that tofu!

SWEETENERS

After everything we've learned about the connection between PCOS and high blood sugar, it makes sense that we should be mindful of our intake of different sweeteners. Even "natural" sweeteners like honey, maple syrup, and agave can spike our blood sugar (which we *really* want to avoid so that we stay clear of a prediabetes diagnosis). But, that doesn't mean we can't have any sweeteners ever. Here are my top sweetener recommendations:

→ Monk fruit

→ Allulose

→ Stevia

→ Erythritol

→ Xylitol

→ Dates (whole, not date syrup)

Use sparingly:

→ Cane sugar (white or brown)

→ Honey

→ Maple syrup

→ Coconut sugar

With those tips, you'll be able to enjoy a sweet tooth craving and keep your best buddy insulin happy and steady.

THE GOAL:
EATING TO BALANCE BLOOD SUGAR

Everything we've covered here—eating your protein, fat, fiber (and even carbs!)—along with getting adequate amounts of micronutrients plus the right doses of antioxidants and anti-inflammatories is *key to eating your way to good health*. When you eat this way and intentionally reduce your sugar intake, you will reduce your blood sugar spikes, support your insulin levels, and help balance and regulate your hormones.

We want to eat to balance our blood sugar. This is the best, simplest, and cheapest way to prevent unwanted PCOS symptoms and the development of chronic lifestyle diseases.

Shifting your diet to include more whole foods and balancing blood sugar will also help you eat yourself to a smaller pants size.

Again, when we aim for balance, we get a great side effect: balanced blood sugar. And when we have balanced blood sugar, that will significantly decrease the up and down of our hormone levels, which causes the unwanted and gnarly symptoms so many of us PCOS warriors face. When our blood sugar is happy, we will have more regular periods, less facial hair, easier weight loss, and even less acne.

The key is consistency. Despite what diet

culture will have us think, there are no bad days. Healthy living is about balance. You can't just give up because you had pizza on a Friday and then did not eat well for a week. You're human. Life happens. If this whole nutrition manual were a class, aim for the B grade instead of the A+.

If you are overwhelmed with *what* exactly you should be eating, that's when I recommend working directly with a dietitian. We can help you do the math to understand what your specific macros, micros, and carb tolerances are. We find these numbers through specific calculations. Through math and science, we will help you:

→ Determine how many calories you need to eat per day and how many of those calories should come directly from carbohydrates, protein, and fat.

→ Determine the exact number of grams of carbohydrates, protein, and fat you should eat each day.

→ Learn how to adjust your carbohydrate intake based on your body signals.

→ Track your macronutrient intake.

These calculations are what every influencer is talking about when they mention micros, macros, and so on! Understanding what yours are can help you reach your weight loss goals faster and with less frustration. However, one word of valuable advice if you decide to work with a dietitian and find out your numbers: Don't get too caught up (and in the weeds) with hitting your macros perfectly every single day! These are targets to aim for, so don't feel too pressured to hit them spot-on all the time. If this process becomes too stressful for you, please use my PCOS plate method.

THE PCOS PLATE METHOD

If you need more help with figuring out how to implement everything I've mentioned here, I have the tool for you! I call it the PCOS plate method.

If you're the kind of person who loves simplicity, you're going to love the PCOS plate method. It's a simple tool that acts as a road map showing you how to portion your meals throughout the day and get your macros for each meal.

The first step of the plate method aims to help you calculate how to divide your calories throughout the day. The amount of calories you're eating is going to depend on your body and your goals, but you should be aiming for your calories to be split roughly like this:

→ 20% = Breakfast

→ 27% = Lunch

→ 27% = Dinner

→ 13% = Snack 1

→ 13% = Snack 2

Yes, 26 percent of your daily calories should come from snacks! Remember, healthy snacks control our blood sugar and cravings throughout the day (just don't forget the protein, ladies!).

Now, we can zoom in on each meal. This is where we picture how we're filling our plate. Your plate should look like this:

→ Half = Low-Starch Vegetables

→ One-Quarter = Protein

→ Less than One-Quarter (Optional) = Complex Carb

→ Leftover (Optional) = Fats

Veggies are *always* the priority because they're chock-full of all the micros we just talked about. It's important to mix these each meal to keep your micro intake diversified, and you can try them raw or baked, sautéed or grilled, or cooked in different ways to keep things interesting. Mix it up with different herbs, spices, and seasoning blends so veggies can stay interesting for you.

You *don't* have to eat meat in every meal to get your portion of protein. This section of your plate could look like eggs, beans, tofu, tempeh, yogurt, or even just a scoop of protein powder mixed into your bevvie of choice.

And when I say "complex" carb, I mean a carb that has *fiber* (think quinoa, brown rice, or farro). But, the complex carb is an optional part of your meal, so this last quarter on your plate could be filled with extra vegetables and protein instead. Your complex carb could also be a starchy vegetable (think butternut squash, potatoes, yams, spaghetti squash, corn, peas, etc.).

The fat portion is also optional, as it's usually already a part of your meal, although you might not have realized it. Because of its invisibility, it's the hardest macro to calculate and visualize on your plate. These fats usually come in the form of butter and oils used while cooking, dressings on your salads, or cheese, nuts, olives, and so on as part of a dish. If you're working on weight management, do your best at minimizing fats and just guesstimate the calorie content in this tricky bugger.

I also recommend making most of your meals at home and limiting yourself to one or two meals out per week. I know many of you will say, "But, Cory, I don't have time after work to cook!" I can't stress enough how important cooking at home is when all the restaurants and fast-food joints in the country are trying to fill us up on all the wrong things. Takeout food is loaded with extra calories, added sugars, empty carbs, more sodium to bloat us, and trans and saturated fats galore! While it might be easy now, taking off the pounds that takeout food will surely bring will be difficult.

YOU DON'T NEED AN EXTREME DIET TO "HEAL" YOUR PCOS

Okay. We *know* what we need to eat to support our bodies. We know what we should ideally avoid. But girl, do you know what we *need* to talk about? All the rampant BS floating around the internet about what diet types PCOS girlies need to follow to heal their symptoms.

One, I hate to be the bearer of bad news, but PCOS is a lifelong condition. No diet, no magical superfood ingredient, and no one supplement is going to cure your PCOS. Yet, there are so many "quick fixes" and diet fads swimming around on Instagram and TikTok that make me crazy.

I'm going to say it again: The main things that are going to help your PCOS are eating a healthy diet filled with protein, fat, and fiber; movement you love; reducing stress; the right targeted supplement protocol; and making sure your hormones are balanced.

Do you know what won't work? Going keto, fasting intermittently, or becoming a vegan. Like, literally, these are myths. There is not one scientific study supporting the idea that these diets work for PCOS women long-term. In fact, these diets hurt us more than they help us! Don't believe me? Let's investigate, shall we?

Keto

As a woman, and especially as a woman who is athletic in any way, the ketogenic diet is a nightmare for your hormones. Ketosis causes a drop in your thyroid hormones, which reduces sex hormone–binding globulin (SHBG). Your ovaries, in turn, pump out more estrogen, and your periods are heavier and longer.

Other research shows ketosis mimics starvation, which triggers the release of the stress hormone cortisol. High circulating cortisol levels suppress the menstrual cycle, so your periods peace out, leaving you susceptible to bone deterioration.

If the ketogenic diet or any other diet is giving you period problems, it's probs not good for you. Pay attention to your cycle and see how it's affected by your diet. Above anything else, make sure you are nourishing your body and your body feels nourished.

And yes, we do have research studies showing the keto diet can be effective when it comes to insulin resistance. However, the attrition rate (how many people leave the study because they simply can't continue it) in these studies is always so high, we're never left with adequate data! The keto diet is so restrictive and hard to maintain; and because we have PCOS for life, we need something that is going to work long-term.

Vegan

Once upon a time, I was a very sad vegan. Like, very sad. I couldn't eat anything at restaurants, I became iron deficient, my period problems got worse, my hair fell out . . . you get the idea. I thought because I was restricting my foods, that my restrictions were going to help my PCOS symptoms. They didn't. My lack of consumption of protein

actually hurt my health and set me back. True story. So, while being vegan can be great for some, it's been my experience that this super-restrictive diet makes it extremely difficult for women to get adequate amounts of iron and protein.

For PCOS ladies, our hormone health and blood sugar balance are *paramount*. When it comes to veganism, it can be hard to even begin to take in enough protein, fat, and fiber to support healthy insulin and glucose levels without overdoing it on carbohydrates.

So, the question I always get is: "Should I go vegan with PCOS?"

In my professional opinion, no. So, does that mean I'm recommending you stop eating lots of plant-based foods? No. Am I telling you to go out there and support factory farming? Also, no. Am I recommending you start eating three marbled steaks a day, every day? Again, noooo. What I am telling you is that you can and should incorporate foods like meat, seafood, and dairy for healthy blood sugar and happy hormones. Your diet should be about balance. Incorporating some meat, seafood, dairy, and eggs in moderation can help support healthy hormone levels, which improve your PCOS symptoms like weight gain, irregular periods, and facial hair.

And, animal-based foods like meat and

fish have tons of healthy nutrients that benefit our PCOS, like zinc, iron, and B vitamins that support hormone regulation.

Intermittent Fasting

Another diet that I'm not a fan of: intermittent fasting. My biggest stink with this diet fad is that we cannot keep our blood sugar levels stable if we are not eating throughout the day. Plus, if you're gorging on huge meals to prepare for that long fast, your blood sugar will spike, and your insulin resistance will only worsen in the long run. In addition, when we do finally get to sit down and enjoy a meal after fasting, we can see increases in binge behavior as our body tries to overcompensate for missing meals earlier.

While men may be able to intermittently fast their little hearts out, for us ladies, it's more complicated than that. We aren't built the same. There's no way around it: Biologically speaking, our bodies are optimized for fertility and reproduction. If our body goes long periods without food, it shuts down our reproductive function.

So what? you may be thinking. Even if you aren't trying to have a kid anytime soon, healthy estrogen and progesterone production are vital to our energy levels, mood, hair, skin, weight, metabolism, digestion,

sleep health, and more. If not done correctly, research shows intermittent fasting may be harmful to our hormones, namely estrogen balance.

Still, if you are curious about the craze, here are some guidelines to consider if you want to try intermittent fasting.

Don't try if you:

→ Have a history of disordered eating.

→ Are pregnant or trying to conceive.

→ Are currently dealing with hormonal issues.

→ Have adrenal issues.

Please stop if:

→ Your period stops or becomes irregular.

→ You start having sleep issues.

→ You notice negative changes in your skin and/or hair.

→ You experience mood swings and/or brain fog.

The bottom line: Do your research and figure out if intermittent fasting is the best thing for your individual body. We're all different; just because something works for that one girl's aunt's cousin's goat's niece, it doesn't mean it's 100 percent perfect for you.

Gluten-Free

The next one I literally am asked one million times a week. "Do I have to become gluten-free to heal my PCOS?" The short answer is no, you do not have to go gluten-free. There are zero scientific studies proving that gluten is bad for your PCOS.

The more complicated answer: There are folks who need to avoid gluten (celiacs), and yes, there may be certain peeps who benefit from removing gluten (non-celiac gluten sensitivity); but studies show this is less than 6 percent of the population! For women with PCOS, this makes up an even smaller number! The rest of us can enjoy high-fiber gluten-containing foods in normal amounts. So, enjoy your flour in moderation, babe!

Dairy-Free

Just like with gluten, there are zero scientific studies proving that dairy is bad for your PCOS. Anyone claiming this on social media is not getting their facts from the research.

However, research *does* show that dairy can exacerbate skin breakouts for some people who are already experiencing acne. So, if cystic acne is an issue for you, I recommend a three-month elimination phase of dairy to see if your acne improves. This does not mean dairy causes acne, but if you already

are prone to this irritating symptom, it may be worth that trial elimination.

If you find that it isn't affecting your acne, then dairy is fine in moderation. It is a great source of protein, calcium, and other nutrients supportive of hormones like B vitamins and zinc. Eating plenty of antioxidants and anti-inflammatories, getting sunshine and fresh air and exercise, and working on stress will help you so much more than singling out dairy (or gluten) and avoiding them like the plague.

A Note on Gluten and Dairy

You may be saying, "But going gluten- and dairy-free changed my life, Cory!" Or you may have heard stories about how others feel totally refreshed after completely eliminating gluten and dairy. And I'm so happy you or your friends feel better!

But honestly, my professional opinion is that the issue probably wasn't the gluten and dairy in the first place. It was all the other nasty things in the ultraprocessed Frankenfoods we eat, most of which contain either gluten or dairy. Think about all those gums, artificial binders, and other junk that are now in our foods. I think it's those things that are disrupting your health. After all, humans have been safely consuming dairy for nearly 10,000 years. Why did everything change? (We started pumping our foods with fake stuff.) Other than this hypothesis, some women with PCOS may see improvements when they eliminate these foods for the following reasons:

1. Suddenly, by cutting out gluten and dairy, we're paying way more attention to ingredient labels, nutrition facts, and what we're eating. Mindfulness will always improve our overall health, especially when it comes to weight loss and inflammation.

2. Now, with these restrictions, so many foods we're used to eating are suddenly off limits. This includes most foods at restaurants! For example, you go out to eat and pretty much the only available item on the menu that follows this protocol is the salad with chicken. This is the best choice anyway for weight loss and blood sugar balance.

3. When we restrict gluten and dairy, we're usually making choices that are lower carb. This allows for progress in the blood sugar department, not the gluten and dairy themselves.

EATING ON THE CHEAP

I don't know what inflation will be like by the time you read this book, but at the time I'm writing, groceries are at an all-time high. Eggs, meat, and everything else are adding up to hundreds of dollars a week for the average family.

Yet, if we want to stay healthy, control our PCOS, and support our hormones, what are we to do?

Here's what not to do: panic. Just because we want to eat well doesn't mean we need to spend more money at the grocery store. Nope. We don't need to buy the million-dollar supplements or the crazy expensive collagen protein powder. We can buy simple ingredients like broccoli, cauliflower, ground turkey, and some good ol' spices and get to work!

Nothing like a good casserole made with some nutrient-dense veggies to calm the wallet and the hormones! If this interests you, there are loads of recipes in the back of this book to support your hormones and your wallet. There are plenty of ways to eat healthy that will move your body in the direction you want.

My main tip: Focus on eating whole foods, and make sure you are cooking the foods you buy. Nothing adds up more than groceries gone to waste.

EATING ON A BUSY SCHEDULE

If you are concerned about time, Imma bust a myth right here: Nobody needs to spend a million hours a week making everything from scratch. That does not make you a worthier person or even a better mom. No, no, no. What we can do is utilize the incredible variety of foods available to us, like canned beans, chickpea pasta, and delicious frozen veggies that support our budgets, our waistlines, and the inadequate twenty-four hours we all have in a day.

But some days, of course, you just can't fit in the time to cook when everything seems to be going to sh*t. You're sick, or you lost your job, or you're traveling, or you just have zero energy. On days like these, remember my rule: Do the best you can with what you've got. The time will come when you can jump back into healthy habits. But if that time is not right now, that's okay. Give yourself grace, get well, and motivate yourself to get back into your groove when you feel ready.

WORTH-IT FOODS

Before we close out, and you go out there and live your best, healthy(ish) life, I want to leave you with one last tip I personally swear by to lose weight and keep my weight under control: worth-it foods.

Worth-it foods are the foods that are worth it. Like, thinking about a life without these foods would bring you to tears. If you've picked up on the numerous Mexican food references throughout this book, you can probably tell my worth-it foods are burritos, nachos, spicy margaritas, and pretty much anything else the rich Mexican culture

offers. If someone told me I could *never* eat a quesadilla again, I'd just quit and cry. A life without nachos is not what I want to have!

So, I came up with worth-it foods to ensure I can eat the foods I *love* instead of those that are meh on my list. For example, I'm not super into kids' cookies (like the ones they have at birthday parties—sugar cookies with all the super bright colored frosting and sprinkles). So, because these cookies are not on my worth-it list, I *just don't eat them*. It's easier for me to pass on them rather than absently eat a few and regret it later because, well, the cookies aren't worth it for me! I'd rather save my calories for something I really, really love. And I don't shame myself when I eat my worth-it foods on occasion. I just enjoy the d*mn burrito.

I personally like this approach better because it makes for more sustainable behavior. Diet culture will have you go all-out and say, "I'm avoiding sugar this month!" but I promise it will backfire, babe. Instead of punishing yourself (and indulging hardcore later), choose your worth-it foods and savor them. Your mental health will thank you for it. If we never make room for worth-it foods and blatantly ignore the fact that we crave them, we fall into a place of restriction and deprivation. We will get to the point where we need sugar, carbs, or other indulgences and we'll overindulge—then feel awful about it. This binge and purge cycle is bad for our mental health. It causes us to lose motivation and abandon our healthy eating, leaving us feeling ashamed of our cravings. It's just not sustainable.

So, let yourself enjoy some of your faves. And really savor them. Trust me, when you get into this intentional practice, you will feel more motivated in the long run to eat healthy-ish (most of the time).

I promise that when you start this way and get out of the binge/purge/black-and-white thinking, your body will have a clearer method of communicating what it needs. And you want this open communication with your body. After all, your body is your best barometer. If you're feeling pain, if your period is irregular, or if you keep getting sick, that is your body trying to communicate to you that something is off. And that means you need to pause, reset, and do what you must to get your body back into balance.

And you will. Because your body is smart. It's powerful. It's capable of profound healing. It wants to be healthy. All you need to do is make good choices, remember your power, and keep your eye on your intention: living a long and healthy life.

MYTH BUSTING

MYTH ONE:
I HAVE TO GO GLUTEN-FREE
WITH PCOS.

Unless you have celiac disease or a gluten sensitivity, you do not have to go gluten-free with PCOS (there is no research supporting a link between gluten and PCOS!).

MYTH TWO:
I SHOULD TRY THE KETO DIET
FOR MY PCOS.

Let me say this: You are a human being. Human beings need carbohydrates. What the keto diet aims to do is eliminate all carbs, so that is a no-go for us, sweeties! The keto diet is way too restrictive and just not sustainable. PCOS warriors need lots and lots of macros, micros, and antioxidants to thrive. Following the keto diet doesn't let us get everything we need.

MYTH THREE:
BUT A VEGAN DIET SHOULD HELP
WITH MY SYMPTOMS, RIGHT?

Any diet restricting the key nutrients we covered in this chapter isn't going to end well when it comes to our general hormone health. Of course, eating more plant-based foods is always a big win, but incorporating meats, seafood, and protein-rich dairy into our diet is beneficial for getting our needed amounts of protein, B vitamins, iron, and omega-3s, which are all crucial for balanced hormones.

THE WRAP-UP

Ooof! This chapter was jam-packed with info. We covered which essential ingredients you need to eat to thrive, how eating in this fashion will support your health, and how eating this way will help you move unwanted pounds off your body.

While I could ramble endlessly here (I mean, I *am* a PCOS dietitian), everything you need to know about eating comes down to one word: balance.

Nobody eats perfectly all the time, and nobody expects you to do the impossible in your life. Eating well and working toward balance mean getting out of the black-and-white thinking that diet culture demands, exploring what feels good for you, and implementing small changes in your eating that can create lasting changes and align with your goals.

Remember: In the long run, eating well is going to be your best protection, medicine, and ingredient for living a long and healthy life.

SUPPORTING YOUR PCOS

The Heroine's Journey

Not too long ago, a girl entered her twenties feeling like a freak. All this weight piled on in college, but she wasn't totally sure *why*. (It didn't help that she never exercised, ate french-fry-stuffed burritos, and chugged beer on the beach on warm California nights, like, *regularly*.) Despite the friends she made at school, she was confused and frustrated by how awful she felt *all the time*. Her period was missing, showed up randomly, and then, poof, vanished, so she did as the doctor told her and got on the Pill. But d*mn, that medication made her weight balloon and her moods made her feel like she was going insane. Desperate to find a solution, she tried a million and one different brands, to no avail.

After years of anxiety, weight gain, and hair loss, this girl found out about a disorder called PCOS *all on her own*, and when she brought it up to her doctor, her doctor confirmed her fears. But, instead of reducing her paranoia that she was broken, all the doctor said as she ended the conversation was "You are going to need significant medical intervention if you ever want to get pregnant."

Dizzy with sadness, she cried. She cried a lot. After some time, though, she was done being sad. Instead of staying in that place of fear and overwhelm, she decided to try.

Inspired by her dad's recent commitment to health after a prediabetes diagnosis, she became a registered dietitian and learned everything there was to learn about PCOS, metabolism, diabetes, and nutrition. (Turns out there was a lot to learn!) She lost the weight and got her period back.

When she turned twenty-seven, she landed what she thought was her dream job as a food service director for a major company. She was the boss! She had a big salary and was leading a team of fifty people . . . and yet, the details of the job became overwhelming. There was so much pressure. It was a commute from hell. Such. Long. Hours. Everything about her "dream job" was making her symptoms worse. More anxiety, mood swings, and weight gain followed her through her daily war with Bay Area traffic. Month after month, she gained pound after pound.

That lifestyle—one that promoted stress—was unsustainable. It felt like her life was falling apart. Her hair was falling out, her period wouldn't stop, and she felt like a freak again. Lost, confused, and hormonal, she quit.

Babes, that girl was me.

At that moment in time, I was burned the f*ck out. I was so overwhelmed that I didn't know what I was going to do.

At the end of my rope, I grabbed on to the one thing I knew would save me: myself. And so, I worked odd jobs (including a stint working as a dietitian at a women's clinic inside a prison to pay the bills) and put every waking free hour I had into opening The Women's Dietitian.

Flash forward years later, I have helped thousands of women conquer the same symptoms I had, get pregnant, and lose all the weight they wanted.

This book, in so many ways, is an accumulation of everything I learned on this wild journey and a summary of all the different ways I've learned to manage—and support—my PCOS and my health.

I wrote this book for you, my PCOS warrior. Cuz, babe, life is hard, but managing your health doesn't have to be. After going on my own hero's journey, I can confidently say that you don't have to be a victim of your PCOS.

There's a different, healthier, sustainable lifestyle out there for you. I know this because I found it for myself. If you want it, too, you can have it.

I promise.

Even if you are in the pits of despair right now with your symptoms—overwhelmed and overworked—and everything in your life seems to be going wrong, I want you to know that it can and will get better. You can reset your life and health with the tools we learned in this book.

And yes, of course, having PCOS sucks and isn't fair and can make us feel awful—but staying in those emotions does not serve you. It doesn't move you forward. What does move you forward is understanding that you have power in your own life. You can make choices that support you, and those choices can and will move the needle toward sustainable health. Cuz, boo thing, you do have more power than you think. You can decide to be your healthiest self.

When I decided I could be my healthiest self, I was able to switch my habits and behaviors. I fed myself food that supported rather than derailed my health. The realization that I could exercise, sleep, eat (pray and love, ha!) my way to PCOS stability was life-changing.

With acceptance of myself and who I really was, I could choose partners and people who supported my journey instead of filling my life with people who didn't under-

stand my symptoms or just didn't care to. All these small choices enabled me to create a new destiny for myself where my health could thrive.

Everything changed once I understood life wasn't happening to me, but I was an active agent in my future. This mindset shift allowed me to see the truth: My PCOS enabled me to take better care of myself. Because I had this diagnosis, I could take active steps to live my healthiest life possible and avoid chronic diseases that plague Americans and kill so many people unnecessarily.

All I had to do was eat healthily (mostly—not all the time), watch my sugar and carb intake to not spike my insulin too much, and learn helpful and actionable ways to consistently de-stress.

Well d*mn. It turns out that with good, consistent, and simple choices, I could lose the weight I wanted, have the babies I dreamed of, and create a family I'm obsessed with. I didn't have to overspend on fancy self-care rituals or even eat super-duper organic food. I could do a face mask from CVS, load up mac and cheese with broccoli and chicken for lunch, have a gorgeous vegetable soup for dinner, and still see remarkable results. And the same is available for you.

It doesn't matter what you see on the internet: Healthy living can be simple, it can be affordable, and it should be accessible. After everything you've read in this book, I hope you feel like it really is doable.

Despite what others will have you think, taking care of your PCOS doesn't have to be this super-confusing, expensive, super-niche thing. You don't have to be vegan, gluten-free, dairy-free, joy-free, or keto to manage your health like a boss. Just make good choices *most of the time.*

Of course, your health journey is never going to be linear. You're going to have good days, and you're going to have days when you just want to hide in your bed with a bowl of raw cookie dough. But you can't give up just because you ate too many cookies one day. You can reset your health at any time, any day of the week. Cuz, girl, you are in charge of your own life, of your own health, and your own outcomes.

And so, in this last part of the book, I want to offer that PCOS can be your power in this complicated life we live. It's definitely mine. My PCOS has made me a stronger woman, ready to face any challenge thrown my way. I never would've found this incredible strength inside of me if I hadn't gone through this journey of figuring out what the hell PCOS was and then conquering it like a bad*ss.

Today, I'm a completely different person from when I first got diagnosed with PCOS. After implementing the lifestyle changes, long-term habits, and mindset makeovers I've offered throughout this book, I can confidently say I live my best life with a beautiful family and symptoms that don't whack me out.

I'm cooking and eating delicious meals that balance my hormones. My cholesterol levels are level. My insulin is steady. I can maintain my weight without dedicating my entire life to counting carbs. My hair has grown back, and my periods, thank the freakin' lord, are regular (most of the time!). I ovulate more often than I don't, and I feel good. I'm sticking to an exercise routine that works for me, and I have a better relationship with stress. Oh, and those people in my life who didn't support my PCOS or care to understand it? Buh bye.

All those results are from everything I've taught in this book. Even though my mom would say otherwise, the truth is I'm not special. I just learned what I needed to learn to achieve sustainable health results. And now, you have all the tools, steps, and knowledge to create the same results in your life. My story can be yours, too.

But I wouldn't be doing my due diligence if I didn't send you off with some PCOS-approved recipes! So, next, you'll find six weeks of delicious recipes that will support your hormones, fertility, waistline, and taste buds. I personally developed these recipes, and, if I do say so myself, they are fire.

With these recipes and meal plans, I am confident that you have everything you need to succeed on your health journey.

With so much love, I send you off into the world with all the information you need to manage your PCOS, live life like a d*mn rock star, and reset your health. Get cooking, remember your worth-it foods, and keep in touch!

THINGS THAT TASTE GOOD

HOW TO USE THIS SECTION

So now that we know basically everything there is to know about how to eat for our PCOS . . . how do we take action on it? Welcome to my PCOS-approved meal plans! These babies were built with your hormones, nutrient needs, and of course taste buds in mind. In this section, you'll find six weeks of meal plans for you to follow! Listen, if you're like me, you love to eat, so don't thumb through here expecting cardboard pancakes or another "baked chicken breast and brown rice" meal. These recipes are inspired from dishes you already love, like gooey chicken parmesan, burgers with crispy sweet potato fries, and mouthwatering pizza, only they've gotten a PCOS-friendly glow up. Each meal plan comes with a variety of breakfast, lunch, dinner, and snack recipes along with a shopping list to make it all easy on you. I hope you enjoy!

Shopping for Specific Amounts

You'll notice the shopping lists give you the specific amount of an ingredient, such as one cup of soy sauce instead of one bottle of soy sauce. This was intentional, so that you could quickly scan your kitchen and see if you happened to have enough of a particular ingredient without having to buy a whole new bottle or package. My hope is that giving you the true measurement in the shopping lists can cut down on overbuying and overspending when putting together your grocery lists for your meal plan.

What's Up with the Five-Day Meal Plan?

Let's be real, no one wants to cook every single meal for themselves (and also family members) seven days a week . . . including ME. I included five instead of seven days in the meal plans so you can exercise some flexibility on the weekends, utilize leftovers, order healthy takeout, and/or plan a fun day or two out. Approaching dietary changes with PCOS requires this type of flexibility so we don't completely burn ourselves out! Feel free to double a recipe or two if you'd like to use leftovers over the weekend and stick to a more structured plan.

Recipes on Repeat

Girl, no one wants to cook an entirely separate meal every single day, three times a day! When it comes to ease, budgetary concerns, and longevity of a "nutrition" plan, leftovers are king! Errr . . . I mean queen, of course. By cooking a dish and spreading it out over multiple meals, we can save time, money, and our precious energy. Learn to love those leftovers!

WEEK 1 — MEAL PLAN

MONDAY

Breakfast: Good Morning Sunshine Smoothie (page 156)

Lunch: Greek Chicken Herb Bowl (page 161)

Dinner: One-Pan Southwest Shrimp and Asparagus (page 159)

TUESDAY

Breakfast: Confetti Egg Muffins (page 157)

Lunch: One-Pan Southwest Shrimp and Asparagus (page 159)

Dinner: Greek Chicken Herb Bowl (page 161)

WEDNESDAY

Breakfast: Good Morning Sunshine Smoothie (page 156)

Lunch: One-Pan Southwest Shrimp and Asparagus (page 159)

Dinner: Egg Roll in a Bowl (page 160)

THURSDAY

Breakfast: Confetti Egg Muffins (page 157)

Lunch: Tuna Salad Lunch Box (page 158)

Dinner: Egg Roll in a Bowl (page 160)

FRIDAY

Breakfast: Confetti Egg Muffins (page 157)

Lunch: Tuna Salad Lunch Box (page 158)

Dinner: Egg Roll in a Bowl (page 160)

WEEK 1 · SHOPPING LIST

PANTRY ITEMS

Extra-virgin olive oil

Olive oil spray

Sesame oil

1½ tablespoons apple cider vinegar

¼ cup chicken or beef bone broth

⅓ cup low-sodium soy sauce

Sea salt

Black pepper

Garlic powder

Red pepper flakes

Italian seasoning

Taco seasoning

Ground cinnamon

PRODUCE

½ cup frozen raspberries

¾ cup fresh raspberries

2 lemons

1 orange

2 medium zucchini

1½ cups grape tomatoes

1 cup baby carrots

1 cup sliced cucumber

1½ pounds asparagus

1 head red cabbage

1 head green cabbage

1 medium carrot

1 red bell pepper

1 cup fresh green beans

2 large yellow onions

2 tablespoons chopped red onion

4 cloves garlic

¼-inch piece fresh ginger

2 tablespoons minced fresh chives

1 bunch cilantro

PROTEINS

2 scoops vanilla protein powder

5 eggs

¼ cup liquid egg whites

8-ounce container feta cheese

⅓ cup plain low-fat Greek yogurt

2 (5-ounce) cans light tuna

1 pound lean ground pork

3 boneless, skinless chicken breasts

1 pound large shrimp

½ cup cooked ham

1 teaspoon sesame seeds

OTHER

2 cups almond milk

¼ cup salted cashews

2 teaspoons ground flaxseed

2 tablespoons cashew or nut butter

3 tablespoons whole milk (can be nondairy)

1 tablespoon monk fruit or allulose
granulated sweetener

¾ cup cooked brown rice

¾ cup cooked tricolor quinoa

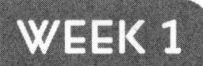

1. ¼ cup salted cashews (or any nut/seed) + ¼ cup berries (any kind)

2. ¾ cup 0% fat plain Greek yogurt mixed with one-half mashed banana and cinnamon

3. 1 Yasso Greek yogurt bar (any flavor)

4. ⅓ cup roasted chickpeas (The Good Bean, Biena Snacks, and Saffron Road are some good brands I suggest)

5. ¼ cup hummus with 1 cup baby carrots, sliced cucumber, or cherry tomatoes

GOOD MORNING SUNSHINE SMOOTHIE

Serves 1
Prep Time: 5 minutes
Calories: 306 per serving
Carbs: 22g per serving

1 cup almond milk
½ cup frozen raspberries
½ fresh orange
1 scoop vanilla protein powder
1 tablespoon cashew or other nut/seed butter
1 teaspoon ground flaxseed
⅛ teaspoon ground cinnamon

Blend all the ingredients together and enjoy!

CONFETTI EGG MUFFINS

Serves 3
Prep Time: 15 minutes
Cook Time: 25 minutes
Calories: 245 per serving
Carbs: 6g per serving

5 eggs
¼ cup egg whites
3 tablespoons whole milk (can be nondairy)
½ red bell pepper, diced
¼ cup crumbled feta cheese
3 tablespoons minced fresh chives
½ cup (heaping) diced cooked ham
⅛ teaspoon sea salt
¼ teaspoon black pepper
¾ cup fresh raspberries, for serving

Preheat the oven to 375°F. Spray a 6-cup muffin pan well with 1 or 2 sprays of olive oil cooking spray.

Crack the eggs into a large mixing bowl and add the egg whites and milk. Whisk until just combined.

Mix in the bell pepper, feta cheese, chives, ham, salt, and pepper.

Fill each muffin cup nearly to the top.

Bake until the eggs are just barely set, 22 to 25 minutes.

Let the muffins cool on a wire rack for 5 minutes, then serve. If you are storing the egg muffins in the fridge or freezer, let them cool for another 5 minutes.

Serve each with ¼ cup fresh raspberries.

TUNA SALAD LUNCH BOX

Serves 2
Prep Time: 10 minutes
Calories: 300 per serving
Carbs: 25g per serving

Two 5-ounce cans light tuna
⅓ cup plain low-fat Greek yogurt
2 tablespoons chopped red onion
Salt and black pepper
1 cup baby carrots
1 cup sliced cucumber
¼ cup salted cashews

In a small bowl, combine the tuna, yogurt, red onion, and salt and pepper to taste.

Serve with the baby carrots and cucumber for dipping with the cashews on the side.

ONE-PAN SOUTHWEST SHRIMP AND ASPARAGUS

Serves 3
Prep Time: 15 minutes
Cook Time: 15 minutes
Calories: 350 per serving
Carbs: 21g per serving

1 pound large shrimp, peeled and deveined
1 tablespoon taco seasoning
3 tablespoons extra-virgin olive oil, divided
¼ cup chicken or beef bone broth
1 tablespoon lemon juice
½ yellow onion, diced
1½ pounds asparagus (1 or 2 bunches), rinsed and trimmed
¾ cup cooked tricolor quinoa

In a medium bowl, combine the shrimp and taco seasoning. Mix well and set aside.

Heat 2 tablespoons of olive oil in a large skillet over medium-high heat. Add the shrimp and cook for 4 to 6 minutes, flipping the shrimp halfway through, until cooked through and no longer pink. Set aside.

In the same skillet (wipe out residual oil and spices if necessary), add the remaining 1 tablespoon olive oil and lower the heat to medium. Add the bone broth and lemon juice and bring to a simmer. Allow the sauce to reduce and thicken a little, then add the onion and asparagus and cook until the asparagus is crisp-tender and the onions are softened, 5 to 7 minutes.

Return the shrimp to the pan. Add the cooked quinoa and warm for 1 to 2 minutes. Remove from the heat and serve.

EGG ROLL IN A BOWL

Serves 3
Prep Time: 15 minutes
Cook Time: 20 minutes
Calories: 360 per serving
Carbs: 9g per serving

1 pound lean ground pork
1 tablespoon sesame oil
4 garlic cloves, minced
¾ tablespoon finely grated fresh ginger
½ yellow onion, diced
½ head red cabbage, shredded
½ head green cabbage, shredded
1 medium carrot, grated
⅓ cup low-sodium soy sauce
1½ tablespoons apple cider vinegar
1 teaspoon sesame seeds
1 tablespoon monk fruit or allulose granulated sweetener
¼ cup cilantro, loosely packed, chopped
¾ cup cooked brown rice

Heat a medium skillet over medium-high heat and add the ground pork. Use a spatula to break it into small pieces, stirring it to cook it through. Cook for 8 to 10 minutes, until no longer pink. Drain any residual grease from the pan.

Add the sesame oil, 3 of the minced cloves of garlic, the ginger, and onion and let them simmer for 1 to 2 minutes, until fragrant.

Add the cabbages, carrot, soy sauce, vinegar, sesame seeds, monk fruit sweetener, and remaining 1 clove of minced garlic to the pan and cook for 4 to 6 minutes, stirring frequently but carefully. The cabbage should be just starting to wilt but not mushy.

Remove from the heat, serve each serving over ¼ cup brown rice, garnish with cilantro, and enjoy!

GREEK CHICKEN HERB BOWLS

Serves 3
Prep Time: 15 minutes
Cook Time: 25 minutes
Calories: 287 per serving
Carbs: 7g per serving

3 boneless, skinless chicken breasts
3 tablespoons extra-virgin olive oil
3 tablespoons Italian seasoning
1 teaspoon garlic powder
Sea salt
Black pepper
2 medium zucchini, sliced into half-moons
1 cup fresh green beans, trimmed
1½ cups grape tomatoes, halved
⅓ large yellow onion, cut into medium half-moons (about ¾ cup)
Juice from 1 lemon
6 tablespoons feta cheese

Preheat the oven to 400°F. Line a sheet pan with parchment paper and grease well.

Place the chicken on the prepared baking pan, arranging on one side of the pan. Brush the chicken on both sides with 1 tablespoon of the olive oil, then season both sides of the chicken with half of the Italian seasoning and half of the garlic powder. Season with salt and pepper. In a large bowl, toss the vegetables with the remaining 2 tablespoons olive oil. Add the remaining Italian seasoning and garlic powder. Toss to coat evenly. Arrange the veggies in a single layer on the other side of the baking pan, making sure they are not mixed with the chicken. Sprinkle the vegetables with salt and pepper to taste.

Drizzle lemon juice over the chicken and veggies. Roast for 20 to 25 minutes, until the veggies are soft and the chicken is cooked through or reaches an internal temperature of 165°F.

Slice the chicken and transfer it to bowls. Fill the rest of the bowls with veggies. Sprinkle each serving with 2 tablespoons feta cheese.

WEEK 2 MEAL PLAN

MONDAY

Breakfast: Blueberry Vanilla Smoothie (page 165)

Lunch: Snack Stack Lunch (page 168)

Dinner: Veggie Cheese Frittata (page 167)

TUESDAY

Breakfast: Savory Oatmeal (page 166)

Lunch: Snack Stack Lunch (page 168)

Dinner: Veggie Cheese Frittata (page 167)

WEDNESDAY

Breakfast: Blueberry Vanilla Smoothie (page 165)

Lunch: Veggie Cheese Frittata (page 167)

Dinner: Lightened-Up Chicken Parmesan (page 169)

THURSDAY

Breakfast: Savory Oatmeal (page 166)

Lunch: Lightened-Up Chicken Parmesan (page 169)

Dinner: Mediterranean Baked Salmon (page 170)

FRIDAY

Breakfast: Blueberry Vanilla Smoothie (page 165)

Lunch: Mediterranean Baked Salmon (page 170)

Dinner: Lightened-Up Chicken Parmesan (page 169)

PANTRY ITEMS

Extra-virgin olive oil

Avocado oil

Olive oil or avocado oil spray

1 cup dry rolled oats

¼ cup almond flour

1 cup cooked brown rice

1 cup vodka pasta sauce

⅓ cup pitted green olives

6 tablespoons nut butter of choice

Sea salt

Black pepper

Paprika

Garlic salt

Garlic powder

Italian seasoning

Ground cinnamon

Ground cumin

PRODUCE

¾ cup frozen blueberries

2 cups fresh blueberries

2 lemons

1 avocado

3 cups fresh arugula

13 cups fresh baby spinach

2 cups fresh curly kale

2 orange bell peppers

2 cups baby carrots

2 whole Roma tomatoes

½ cup cherry tomatoes

3 medium-large carrots

1 red onion

2 cloves garlic

1 bunch fresh dill

PROTEINS

3 scoops vanilla protein powder

10 eggs

¾ cup shredded cheddar cheese

½ cup + 2 tablespoons grated Parmesan cheese

3 slices provolone cheese

2 fresh salmon fillets

3 medium boneless, skinless chicken breasts

20 slices light Italian dry salami

OTHER

3 cups unsweetened almond milk

¼ cup whole milk (can also be nondairy)

3 tablespoons chia seeds

3 tablespoons walnuts or other nut/seed

4 tablespoons tzatziki or hummus

1. Brown rice cake topped with 2 tablespoons hummus and sliced cucumber/cherry tomatoes with salt and pepper or topped with 1 tablespoon melted nut butter and cinnamon

2. 1 ounce (about 10) roasted, salted macadamia nuts with ¼ cup fresh berries

3. Quesadilla: 2 small corn tortillas with ¼ cup shredded melted cheese and salsa inside

4. Think! protein bar, Love Good Fats protein bar, or Rx Bar—any flavor

5. Celery sticks with 2 tablespoons nut or seed butter of choice and cinnamon

BLUEBERRY VANILLA SMOOTHIE

Serves 1
Prep Time: 5 minutes
Calories: 400 per serving
Carbs: 22g per serving

1 cup unsweetened plain or vanilla almond milk
¼ cup frozen blueberries
1 scoop vanilla protein powder
1 cup fresh baby spinach
2 tablespoons cashew or other nut/seed butter
1 tablespoon chia seeds
Pinch of cinnamon
Pinch of sea salt

In a blender, combine the milk, blueberries, protein powder, baby spinach, cashew butter, chia seeds, cinnamon, and sea salt and blend until smooth.

SAVORY OATMEAL

Serves 1
Prep Time: 5 minutes
Cook Time: 10 minutes
Calories: 430 per serving
Carbs: 35g per serving

1 cup water
½ cup rolled oats
Salt
Pinch of garlic powder
1 teaspoon extra-virgin olive oil
2 eggs
1 cup fresh baby spinach, loosely packed
¼ avocado, sliced
2 tablespoons grated Parmesan cheese
Black pepper

In a medium saucepan, bring the water to a boil over medium-high heat. Add the oats, a pinch of salt, and the garlic powder and cover. Lower the heat to a simmer, and cook for 5 to 6 minutes, until most of the water is absorbed. Set aside.

In a small skillet over medium heat, heat the olive oil for 30 seconds. Crack in both eggs and cook until the whites are set and the yolks are runny, 2 to 3 minutes. Season with salt and remove from the heat. Or you can make 2 scrambled eggs instead. While the pan is still hot, add the spinach and cook until wilted, about 1 minute.

Place the oatmeal in a serving bowl. Add the fried eggs, spinach, avocado, Parmesan, and a sprinkle of pepper. Serve warm and enjoy!

VEGGIE CHEESE FRITTATA

Serves 3
Prep Time: 10 minutes
Cook Time: 18 minutes
Calories: 375 per serving
Carbs: 5g per serving

5 eggs
¼ cup whole milk (can also be nondairy)
½ teaspoon sea salt, plus more for finishing
¼ teaspoon black pepper, plus more for finishing
¾ cup shredded cheddar cheese
¼ cup grated Parmesan cheese
½ cup cherry tomatoes, halved
½ orange bell pepper, diced
2 cups loosely packed chopped fresh curly kale
3 cups fresh arugula, loosely packed
Extra-virgin olive oil
3 tablespoons walnuts or other nut/seed
1 lemon

Preheat the oven to 400°F.

In a medium bowl, whisk the eggs, milk, ½ teaspoon salt, and ¼ teaspoon pepper until smooth. Mix in the cheeses, tomatoes, bell pepper, and kale.

Grease a medium baking dish (Pyrex or cast iron work well). Pour the mixture into the dish and bake for 15 to 18 minutes, until the edges are set, the middle still has a very slight jiggle when you shake it, and the top is lightly browned.

Cut into three portions and serve over a bed of arugula dressed with a little olive oil, salt and pepper, 1 tablespoon walnuts each, and a squeeze of fresh lemon juice.

SNACK STACK LUNCH

Serves 1
Prep Time: 5 minutes
Calories: 365 per serving
Carbs: 30g per serving

10 slices light Italian dry salami or 4 ounces deli sliced turkey
½ avocado, sliced
1 cup blueberries
1 cup baby carrots
2 tablespoons tzatziki or hummus

Enjoy!

LIGHTENED-UP CHICKEN PARMESAN

Serves 3
Prep Time: 15 minutes
Cook Time: 25 minutes
Calories: 425 per serving
Carbs: 18g per serving

1 egg
¼ cup almond flour
¼ cup grated Parmesan cheese
1 teaspoon garlic salt
1 teaspoon Italian seasoning
3 medium boneless, skinless chicken breasts, sliced in half lengthwise
6 cups baby spinach
1 cup vodka sauce
3 slices provolone cheese

Preheat the oven to 400°F. Line a baking sheet with parchment paper.

In a shallow bowl, whisk the egg.

In another shallow bowl, mix together the almond flour, Parmesan, garlic salt, and Italian seasoning.

Dip each piece of chicken in the egg mixture, flipping it to cover both sides, then transfer it to the almond flour mixture. Cover the chicken completely with the almond flour mixture, making certain all sides are coated. Repeat with the remaining pieces of chicken.

Transfer the coated chicken pieces to the prepared baking sheet. Bake for 20 minutes, remove from the oven, then scatter the baby spinach all over the pan.

Spoon one-third of the vodka sauce over each piece of chicken and arrange the provolone slices on top. Broil until the cheese is bubbly and lightly browned.

MEDITERRANEAN BAKED SALMON

Serves 2
Prep Time: 20 minutes
Cook Time: 35 minutes
Calories: 415 per serving
Carbs: 33g per serving

2 fresh salmon fillets
Sea salt and black pepper
2 tablespoons avocado oil
Juice of ½ lemon
2 cloves garlic, minced
½ teaspoon Italian seasoning
½ teaspoon paprika
½ teaspoon garlic powder
2 whole Roma tomatoes, thinly sliced
1 orange bell pepper, thinly sliced
½ red onion, thinly sliced
⅓ cups pitted green olives
3 medium-large carrots, sliced into spears
1 tablespoon olive oil
2 tablespoons minced fresh dill
Pinch each of salt, black pepper, ground cumin, paprika, and garlic powder
1 cup cooked brown rice

Preheat the oven to 425°F. Cover two sheet pans with parchment paper.

Season both sides of the salmon with salt and pepper and set aside.

In a small mixing bowl, whisk together the avocado oil, lemon juice, garlic, Italian seasoning, paprika, and garlic powder. Set aside.

Fold two large pieces of parchment paper down the middle to make two halves.

Evenly distribute the tomatoes, bell pepper, onion, and olives in the bottom of each piece of parchment paper. Place one salmon fillet on top of each. Drizzle half of the avocado oil mixture over each packet. Fold the top half of the parchment paper over the bottom half, then roll up the edges around the salmon and vegetables to create a "packet." Repeat for the remaining packet. Place both salmon packets on one of the prepared baking pans.

In a medium bowl, toss the carrots, olive oil, dill, and spices and spread them on the other prepared baking pan.

Place both baking pans in the oven. Bake the salmon for 12 to 15 minutes, until fully cooked and the salmon flakes easily with a fork. Turn down the oven temperature to 375°F and bake the carrots for 15 to 20 minutes more, until fork-tender.

Serve the carrots with the salmon packets and ½ cup brown rice per serving.

WEEK 3 MEAL PLAN

MONDAY

Breakfast: Portobello Baked Eggs (page 175)

Lunch: Sesame Cashew Wrap (page 177)

Dinner: Pesto Sheet Pan Chicken and Veggies (page 181)

TUESDAY

Breakfast: Mango Lime Chia Mousse (page 176)

Lunch: Sesame Cashew Wrap (page 177)

Dinner: Pesto Sheet Pan Chicken and Veggies (page 181)

WEDNESDAY

Breakfast: Mango Lime Chia Mousse (page 176)

Lunch: Pesto Sheet Pan Chicken and Veggies (page 181)

Dinner: Sesame Cashew Wrap (page 177)

THURSDAY

Breakfast: Portobello Baked Eggs (page 175)

Lunch: Salmon Burger and Tangy Slaw (page 178)

Dinner: Garlic Butter Pork Skillet (page 180)

FRIDAY

Breakfast: Mango Lime Chia Mousse (page 176)

Lunch: Salmon Burger and Tangy Slaw (page 178)

Dinner: Garlic Butter Pork Skillet (page 180)

SHOPPING LIST

PANTRY ITEMS

Extra-virgin olive oil
Avocado oil
Sesame oil
1 tablespoon rice wine vinegar
1½ tablespoons apple cider vinegar
⅓ cup + 1 tablespoon low-sodium soy sauce
3 tablespoons liquid sweetener of choice
1 tablespoon granulated allulose or monk
 fruit sweetener
½ teaspoon pure vanilla extract
Red pepper flakes

⅓ cup oat flour
One 15-ounce can black beans
3 large low-carb burrito tortillas
Sea salt
Black pepper
Garlic powder
Onion powder
Paprika
Ground turmeric
Ground cinnamon

PRODUCE

2 cups mango, fresh or frozen
2 medium tangerines
1 lemon
2 limes
2 avocados
1 medium carrot
4 portobello mushrooms
1 head cauliflower
One 14-ounce bag fresh riced cauliflower

Two 8-ounce bags tricolor coleslaw
1 small cucumber
1 russet potato
1 small shallot
2 bunches green onions
2 cloves fresh garlic
½ cup + 1 tablespoon fresh cilantro
¼ cup minced fresh dill
2 tablespoons chopped fresh chives

PROTEINS

3 scoops vanilla protein powder
5 eggs
¼ cup shredded Parmesan cheese
½ cup plain low-fat Greek yogurt
½ pound lean ground pork

3 skin-on, bone-in chicken thighs
1 rotisserie chicken
10 ounces canned salmon
½ cup cooked shelled edamame

OTHER

2 cups unsweetened almond milk
2 tablespoons unsalted butter
¼ cup roasted cashews

½ cup chia seeds
¼ cup jarred pesto

1. 1 package roasted seaweed snacks + ¼ sliced avocado + handful of sprouts; wrap the slices of avocado and sprouts in seaweed.

2. 1 cup Magic Spoon cereal with ¾ cup unsweetened plant-based milk, or ¾ cup Catalina Crunch cereal with 1 cup unsweetened plant-based milk

3. 2 tablespoons dark chocolate chips + 2 tablespoons roasted nuts or pumpkin/sunflower seeds

4. 1 hard-boiled egg + 2 ounces salami or cheese

5. ½ cup whole milk cottage cheese + ¼ cup chopped fresh or frozen/thawed pineapple

PORTOBELLO BAKED EGGS

Serves 1
Prep Time: 5 minutes
Cook Time: 22 minutes
Calories: 366 per serving
Carbs: 30g per serving

2 portobello mushrooms, peeled and stemmed
2 eggs
Pinch of sea salt and black pepper
2 tablespoons shredded Parmesan cheese
1 medium tangerine
½ avocado

Preheat the oven to 400°F.

Place the portobello mushrooms on a baking pan, stem side up.

Carefully crack an egg into each mushroom. Season with the salt and pepper and bake for 18 to 22 minutes, until the whites of the eggs are cooked through and the yolks are set. Sprinkle 1 tablespoon of Parmesan over each egg/mushroom before serving and serve with 1 medium tangerine and ½ avocado. Enjoy warm!

MANGO LIME CHIA MOUSSE

Serves 3
Prep Time: 10 minutes
Calories: 352 per serving
Carbs: 24g per serving

2 cups unsweetened plain almond milk
3 scoops vanilla protein powder
½ cup chia seeds
½ teaspoon pure vanilla extract
3 tablespoons liquid sweetener of choice (allulose, monk fruit, or sugar-free maple syrup)
2 cups chopped mango (thawed, if frozen)
2 tablespoons fresh lime juice

In a large bowl, mix the milk, protein powder, chia seeds, vanilla, and sweetener until thoroughly combined. Place in the fridge to chill for at least 4 hours or overnight.

Once the mixture has thickened into a pudding-like consistency, place it in a blender along with the mango and lime juice. Blend well. Feel free to omit this step if you'd rather not blend it.

Pour the mousse into a glass, bowl, or jar for serving. The mixture can be kept in the fridge for a few days if needed and is best enjoyed cold.

SESAME CASHEW WRAP

Serves 3
Prep Time: 20 minutes
Cook Time: 10 minutes
Calories: 495 per serving
Carbs: 40g per serving

Dressing

2 tablespoons sesame oil
1 tablespoon avocado oil
1 garlic clove, minced
1 tablespoon rice wine vinegar
1 tablespoon low-sodium soy sauce
1 tablespoon granulated monk fruit or allulose sweetener

Salad

2 cups tricolor coleslaw
1 small cucumber, peeled and diced
1 medium carrot, grated
½ cup fresh cilantro, chopped
½ cup sliced green onion, green portion only
½ cup cooked shelled edamame
¼ cup roasted cashew halves
2 cups diced rotisserie chicken
3 large low-carb burrito tortillas

To make the dressing: In a small bowl, whisk the sesame oil, avocado oil, garlic, vinegar, soy sauce, and monk fruit or allulose sweetener until smooth.

To make the salad: In a large bowl, combine the coleslaw, cucumber, carrot, cilantro, green onion, edamame, cashews, and chicken. Toss all the salad ingredients together, drizzle with the dressing, and mix to combine.

Lay a tortilla flat on a cutting board and scoop one-third of the salad mixture on top. Roll into a burrito shape and repeat for each wrap.

SALMON BURGER AND TANGY SLAW

Serves 2
Prep Time: 15 minutes
Cook Time: 10 minutes
Calories: 410 per serving
Carbs: 11g per serving

Salmon Burger

10 ounces canned salmon, drained and flaked with a fork
1 egg
⅓ cup oat flour
½ teaspoon sea salt
2 tablespoons minced fresh dill
2 tablespoons sliced fresh green onion, green portion only
¼ teaspoon garlic powder
¼ teaspoon onion powder
⅛ teaspoon paprika
⅛ teaspoon ground black pepper
1 tablespoon lemon juice
1 tablespoon extra-virgin olive oil

Tangy Slaw

4 cups tricolor coleslaw
½ cup plain low-fat Greek yogurt
½ teaspoon salt
2 tablespoons chopped fresh chives
2 tablespoons minced fresh dill
1 small garlic clove, minced
1 to 2 tablespoons avocado oil
1 to 1½ tablespoons apple cider vinegar, or more to taste
½ avocado for serving

To make the salmon burgers: In a large bowl, mix together the salmon, egg, oat flour, salt, the dill, green onion, garlic powder, onion powder, paprika, pepper, and lemon juice and form four equal patties. If needed, add more oat flour to make them hold together better. In a large nonstick skillet, heat the olive oil over medium heat. Cook the burgers for 4 to 6 minutes, flipping halfway in between, until crispy. Set aside.

To make the slaw: In a medium bowl, mix together the coleslaw, yogurt, salt, chives, dill, garlic, avocado oil, and vinegar.

Serve the salmon burgers on a bed of the tangy slaw with ¼ sliced avocado for each serving.

GARLIC BUTTER PORK SKILLET

Serves 2
Prep Time: 10 minutes
Cook Time: 20 minutes
Calories: 415 per serving
Carbs: 25g per serving

1 tablespoon sesame oil
4 cups fresh riced cauliflower
¼ teaspoon ground turmeric
Sea salt and black pepper
2 tablespoons unsalted butter
½ pound lean ground pork
1 tablespoon minced garlic
⅛ teaspoon red pepper flakes
⅓ cup low-sodium soy sauce
1 tablespoon minced fresh cilantro
½ cup canned black beans, drained and rinsed

In a large skillet over medium heat, warm the sesame oil. Sauté the riced cauliflower for 7 to 10 minutes, until slightly tender. Season with the turmeric and salt and pepper to taste. Remove the cauliflower "rice" to a separate bowl.

In the same skillet (clean out if needed), melt the butter and cook the ground pork until it's no longer pink, 7 to 8 minutes. Add the garlic, red pepper flakes, and soy sauce and cook for 2 more minutes, stirring frequently.

Return the cauliflower rice to the skillet and mix it into the pork. Sprinkle with the cilantro. Serve with ¼ cup black beans per serving.

PESTO SHEET PAN CHICKEN AND VEGGIES

Serves 3
Prep Time: 20 minutes
Cook Time: 45 minutes
Calories: 450 per serving
Carbs: 25 per serving

1 head cauliflower, cut into 1-inch pieces
1 russet potato, cut into 1-inch pieces
1 tablespoon extra-virgin olive oil
½ small lemon, juiced
1 small shallot, minced
½ teaspoon sea salt
⅛ teaspoon ground black pepper
3 skin-on, bone-in chicken thighs
¼ cup jarred pesto

Preheat the oven to 425°F. Cover a rimmed baking sheet with parchment paper.

Place the cauliflower and potato on the baking sheet and toss with the olive oil, lemon juice, shallot, salt, and pepper.

Nestle the chicken skin side up on the baking sheet with the cauliflower and potatoes.

Roast for 40 to 45 minutes, until the chicken reaches an internal temperature of 165°F. Stir the pan halfway through.

Serve the sheet pan topped with the pesto.

WEEK 4 MEAL PLANS

MONDAY

Breakfast: Loaded Smoked Salmon Toast (page 185)

Lunch: Chicken Ranch Wrap (page 187)

Dinner: Zesty Burrito Bowl (page 190)

TUESDAY

Breakfast: Apple Pie Yogurt Bowl (page 186)

Lunch: Zesty Burrito Bowl (page 190)

Dinner: Zucchini Pizza Bites (page 189)

WEDNESDAY

Breakfast: Loaded Smoked Salmon Toast (page 185)

Lunch: Chicken Ranch Wrap (page 187)

Dinner: Zucchini Pizza Bites (page 189)

THURSDAY

Breakfast: Apple Pie Yogurt Bowl (page 186)

Lunch: Zesty Burrito Bowl (page 190)

Dinner: Greek Pita (page 188)

FRIDAY

Breakfast: Apple Pie Yogurt Bowl (page 186)

Lunch: Greek Pita (page 188)

Dinner: Zucchini Pizza Bites (page 189)

PANTRY ITEMS

Extra-virgin olive oil
Avocado oil
Olive oil spray
1 package taco seasoning
6 tablespoons salsa
Sea salt
Black pepper

Ground cinnamon
½ cup no-sugar-added marinara sauce
2 large low-carb tortillas
2 slices whole-grain bread
2 whole-wheat pitas
6 tablespoons unsalted creamy cashew
  butter

PRODUCE

2 green apples
1 cup fresh blueberries
4 pieces romaine lettuce
6 ounces fresh curly kale
2 cups fresh baby spinach, loosely packed
3 cups fresh riced cauliflower
2 cups grape tomatoes
1 beefsteak tomato
2 cups crudité vegetables (can be one or a
  mix of snap peas, baby carrots, and
  grape tomatoes)

3 large zucchinis
1 cup corn kernels, fresh or frozen
Fresh cilantro
1 cup fresh arugula, loosely packed
1 bunch fresh basil
¼ cup diced red onion
1 avocado

PROTEINS

6 eggs
1½ cups shredded mozzarella cheese
⅓ cup crumbled feta cheese
3 tablespoons shredded cheddar cheese
3 cups plain Greek yogurt

1 rotisserie chicken
¾ pound ground chicken
6 ounces smoked salmon
1 cup uncured nitrate/nitrite-free pepperoni
¾ cup black beans

OTHER

2 tablespoons whole milk
2 tablespoons cream cheese
3 tablespoons sour cream

⅓ cup plus 2 tablespoons ranch dressing
2 tablespoons pumpkin seeds/pepitas

PCOS-FRIENDLY SNACKS

1. 2 Roma tomatoes, sliced and sprinkled with ¼ cup crumbled feta cheese and a sprinkle of salt and pepper

2. 1 peach, sliced and drizzled with 1 teaspoon honey, a dash of cinnamon, and chopped fresh mint (optional)

3. 1 ounce Skinny Dipped nuts, any flavor

4. Celery sticks smeared with 2 tablespoons salted, roasted almond butter

5. ¼ cup garlic hummus + ½ cup whole-grain crackers (like Mary's Gone Crackers, Flackers, and Simple Mills)

LOADED SMOKED SALMON TOAST

Serves 1
Prep Time: 5 minutes
Calories: 378 per serving
Carbs: 31g per serving

1 slice whole-grain bread (at least 3g fiber per slice)
1 tablespoon cream cheese, or ¼ sliced avocado, or
    1 tablespoon hummus
3 ounces smoked salmon
½ cup fresh arugula, loosely packed
1 tablespoon pumpkin seeds/pepitas (sunflower seeds or pistachios
    work, too)
Freshly ground black pepper
½ cup fresh blueberries

Toast the bread. Spread the cream cheese on the toast, add the salmon, and top with the arugula. Sprinkle with the pumpkin seeds and a pinch of black pepper.

Serve the toast with the blueberries.

APPLE PIE YOGURT BOWL

Serves 1
Prep Time: 5 minutes
Cook Time: 3 to 4 minutes
Calories: 415 per serving
Carbs: 25g per serving

½ green apple, chopped
A couple sprinkles of cinnamon
1 cup plain Greek yogurt
2 tablespoons unsalted creamy cashew butter (or other nut/seed butter)
Sprinkle of sea salt

Sprinkle the apples with some cinnamon and place in a microwave-safe bowl. Microwave for 3 to 4 minutes, until tender. You can also heat the apples on the stovetop in a small skillet over medium heat until tender.

Into a small bowl, spoon the yogurt, drizzle it with the cashew butter, top with the apples, a sprinkle of salt, and more cinnamon. If needed, heat the cashew butter in the microwave for 10 to 20 seconds, until melted.

CHICKEN RANCH WRAPS

Serves 2
Prep Time: 10 minutes
Cook Time: 10 minutes
Calories: 430 per serving
Carbs: 27g per serving

2 cups shredded rotisserie chicken
⅓ cup plus 2 tablespoons ranch dressing (I like Primal Foods and Chosen)
½ avocado, diced
2 large low-carb burrito tortillas (I like Carb Balance, Ole Extreme, or FlatOut)
4 pieces romaine lettuce
4 slices beefsteak tomato
2 cups crudité vegetables (I like a mix of snap peas, baby carrots, and grape tomatoes)

In a medium bowl, combine the chicken, ⅓ cup of the ranch dressing, and the avocado.

Lay a tortilla flat on a cutting board and place 2 lettuce leaves and 2 tomato slices on top. Scoop half of the chicken mixture on top. Roll into a burrito shape, and repeat for each wrap.

Enjoy each wrap with 1 cup of crudité veggies and 1 tablespoon of the remaining dressing for dipping. Slice in half and serve.

GREEK PITA

Serves 2
Prep Time: 3 minutes
Cook Time: 10 minutes
Calories: 457 per serving
Carbs: 25g per serving

6 eggs
2 tablespoons whole milk (can be nondairy)
¼ teaspoon sea salt
⅛ teaspoon freshly ground black pepper
Olive oil spray
6 ounces curly kale
1 cup grape tomatoes, halved
⅓ cup crumbled feta cheese
2 whole-wheat pitas

In a large bowl, whisk the eggs, milk, salt, and pepper to combine and set aside.

Spray a large nonstick skillet with olive oil spray and heat over medium heat. Add the kale and toss continuously until wilted, about 3 minutes.

Lower the heat to medium-low and pour in the egg mixture. Scramble until the eggs are just set, 4 to 6 minutes.

Remove the pan from the heat and stir in the tomatoes and feta. Divide the mixture in half and stuff each of the 2 pitas.

ZUCCHINI PIZZA BITES

Serves 3
Prep Time: 12 minutes
Cook Time: 15 minutes
Calories: 410 per serving
Carbs: 7g per serving

3 large zucchini, sliced into ¼-inch rounds
Olive oil spray
Sea salt and black pepper
½ cup no-sugar-added marinara sauce (I like Primal Kitchen, Rao's, or Yo Mama's)
1½ cups shredded mozzarella cheese
1 cup uncured nitrate/nitrite-free pepperoni
¼ cup diced red onion
¼ cup chopped fresh basil for garnish

Preheat the oven to broil.

Place zucchini in a single layer on a parchment-lined baking sheet, spray with olive oil spray, and sprinkle with salt and pepper. Broil for 2 minutes on each side. Remove from the oven and turn down the heat to 400°F.

Cover the zucchini slices with the marinara sauce, then layer with the cheese, pepperoni, and diced red onion.

Bake for 8 to 10 minutes, until the cheese is melted and starting to brown and the zucchini is fork-tender. Garnish with the basil and serve warm!

ZESTY BURRITO BOWL

Serves 3
Prep Time: 15 minutes
Cook Time: 20 minutes
Calories: 355 per serving
Carbs: 25g per serving

¾ pound ground chicken
2 tablespoons taco seasoning, divided
1 tablespoon avocado oil
¾ cup black beans
1 cup grape tomatoes
2 cups baby spinach, loosely packed
1 cup corn kernels (can be fresh or frozen and thawed)
3 cups fresh riced cauliflower
3 pinches of chopped fresh cilantro
3 tablespoons shredded cheddar cheese
3 tablespoons sour cream, or 2 to 3 slices avocado
6 tablespoons salsa

In a large nonstick skillet over medium heat, sprinkle the ground chicken with 1 tablespoon of the taco seasoning. Brown the meat, breaking it apart with a wooden spoon until completely cooked, 8 to 10 minutes. Remove the chicken from the heat and set aside.

To the same pan, add the avocado oil and sauté the black beans, grape tomatoes, spinach, corn, and riced cauliflower along with the remaining 1 tablespoon taco seasoning. Cook for 5 to 7 minutes, until the veggies start to soften. Return the chicken to the skillet and reheat while stirring for 1 minute.

Scoop one-third of the meat mixture into a serving bowl, add a pinch of cilantro, 1 tablespoon of cheese, 1 tablespoon of sour cream, and 2 tablespoons of salsa. Repeat for the remaining two servings.

WEEK 5 MEAL PLANS

MONDAY

Breakfast: Pumpkin Pie Yogurt (page 195)

Lunch: Greek Cottage Cheese Bowl (page 196)

Dinner: Veggie Cheese Frittata (page 200)

TUESDAY

Breakfast: Carrot Cake Overnight Oats (page 194)

Lunch: Veggie Cheese Frittata (page 200)

Dinner: Peanut Tofu Bowl (page 198)

WEDNESDAY

Breakfast: Pumpkin Pie Yogurt (page 195)

Lunch: Peanut Tofu Bowl (page 198)

Dinner: Sheet Pan Chicken (page 197)

THURSDAY

Breakfast: Carrot Cake Overnight Oats (page 194)

Lunch: Sheet Pan Chicken (page 197)

Dinner: Greek Cottage Cheese Bowl (page 196)

FRIDAY

Breakfast: Pumpkin Pie Yogurt (page 195)

Lunch: Veggie Cheese Frittata (page 200)

Dinner: Sheet Pan Chicken (page 197)

PANTRY ITEMS

Extra-virgin olive oil
Low-sodium soy sauce
Rice vinegar
2 tablespoons monk fruit or allulose
    granulated sweetener
1 tablespoon sriracha
½ cup peanut butter
3 tablespoons almond butter
3 tablespoons walnuts
2 tablespoons pistachios
1½ tablespoons pumpkin seeds

1 tablespoon chia seeds
1 tablespoon ground flaxseed
½ cup rolled oats
¾ cup canned pumpkin
Sea salt
Black pepper
Ground cinnamon
Pumpkin pie spice
Pure vanilla extract
Garlic powder
Everything bagel seasoning

PRODUCE

1 banana
2 lemons
1 lime
16-ounce bag fresh arugula
16-ounce bag fresh baby spinach
½ cup cherry tomatoes
½ cup grape tomatoes
½ cup chopped Persian cucumbers
1 orange bell pepper

1½ cups small fingerling potatoes
8 medium carrots
1 large head broccoli
1 large yellow onion
1 red onion
2 tablespoons fresh dill
2 tablespoons fresh thyme
4 tablespoons chopped, pitted Kalamata
    olives

PROTEINS

5 eggs
⅔ cup almond milk
¼ cup whole milk
3¼ cups plain low-fat Greek yogurt
2 cups whole-milk cottage cheese

¾ cup shredded cheddar cheese
¼ cup grated Parmesan cheese
3 large skin-on, bone-in chicken thighs
One 14-ounce package firm tofu

1. Mashed avocado with everything bagel seasoning

2. 2 ounces roasted chickpeas

3. Celery sticks with 2 tablespoons nut/seed butter of choice and cinnamon

4. Think! protein bar, Love Good Fats protein bar, or Rx Bar—any flavor

5. Berry Yogurt Bark (page 201)

CARROT CAKE OVERNIGHT OATS

Serves 2
Prep Time: 5 minutes
Calories: 275 per serving
Carbs: 31.5g per serving

⅔ cup unsweetened almond milk (or choice of milk)
½ cup rolled oats
½ cup shredded carrots
½ banana
½ teaspoon ground cinnamon
¼ teaspoon pure vanilla extract
1 tablespoon ground flaxseed
1 cup plain low-fat Greek yogurt

In a large bowl, combine the milk, oats, carrots, banana, cinnamon, vanilla, ground flaxseed, and yogurt. Mix all together, distribute between two jars with lids, and refrigerate overnight.

Enjoy right out of the fridge or heat over the stove or in the microwave until warmed through!

PUMPKIN PIE YOGURT

Serves 1
Prep Time: 5 minutes
Calories: 275 per serving
Carbs: 16g per serving

¾ cup plain low-fat Greek yogurt
¼ cup canned pumpkin
¼ teaspoon ground cinnamon
¼ teaspoon pumpkin pie spice
½ tablespoon pumpkin seeds
1 teaspoon chia seeds
1 tablespoon almond butter

In a medium bowl, combine the yogurt, pumpkin, cinnamon, and pumpkin pie spice. Stir well and top with the pumpkin seeds, chia seeds, and almond butter.

GREEK COTTAGE CHEESE BOWL

Serves 1
Prep Time: 10 minutes
Calories: 310 per serving
Carbs: 20g per serving

1 cup whole-milk cottage cheese
⅛ teaspoon garlic powder
½ cup chopped Persian cucumbers
2 tablespoons thinly sliced red onion
½ cup grape tomatoes, halved
¼ fresh orange bell pepper, diced
2 tablespoons pitted, chopped Kalamata olives
1 tablespoon minced fresh dill
1 tablespoon pistachios
Pinch of everything bagel seasoning

In a small bowl, mix together the cottage cheese and garlic powder. Top with the cucumbers, red onion, grape tomatoes, bell pepper, and olives. Sprinkle with the dill and pistachios and season with the everything bagel seasoning.

SHEET PAN CHICKEN

Serves 3
Prep Time: 10 minutes
Cook Time: 10 minutes
Calories: 400 per serving
Carbs: 30g per serving

6 medium-large carrots, peeled and trimmed
1 large yellow onion, chopped
1½ cups small fingerling potatoes, halved
2 tablespoons extra-virgin olive oil, divided
3 large skin-on, bone-in chicken thighs
2 tablespoons fresh thyme, minced
½ teaspoon sea salt
¼ teaspoon black pepper

Preheat the oven to 425°F and line a baking sheet with parchment paper.

Arrange the carrots and onion on one side of the baking sheet and place the potatoes on the other.

Drizzle 1 tablespoon of the olive oil over the veggies and potatoes.

Rub each chicken thigh with the remaining 1 tablespoon olive oil. Sprinkle the entire pan with the thyme, salt, and pepper. Place the chicken on the baking sheet with the vegetables and potatoes. Roast the entire pan for 20 to 30 minutes, until the chicken skin is golden and the carrots are fork-tender. Test the potatoes and, if needed, move the cooked carrots and chicken onto a serving platter and continue cooking the potatoes until fork-tender (about 10 minutes more).

Divide the chicken, veggies, and potatoes into three servings.

PEANUT TOFU BOWL

Serves 2
Prep Time: 1 hour 15 minutes
Cook Time: 30 minutes
Calories: 435 per serving
Carbs: 23g per serving

Peanut Sauce

½ cup peanut butter
Juice from 1 fresh lime
3 tablespoons low-sodium soy sauce
1 tablespoon rice vinegar
1 tablespoon sriracha
2 tablespoons monk fruit or allulose granulated sweetener

Tofu

One 14-ounce package firm tofu, pressed, drained, and
   chopped into ½-inch cubes

Roasted Broccoli

1 large head broccoli, cut into florets
2 tablespoons olive oil
Pinch of garlic powder
Sea salt and black pepper
½ fresh lemon

To make the peanut sauce: In a medium bowl, whisk the peanut butter, lime juice, soy sauce, vinegar, sriracha, and sweetener until smooth. Add hot water 2 tablespoons at a time if it's too thick.

Carefully add the tofu cubes to the bowl of peanut sauce and toss to coat. Let the tofu marinate in a covered container in the fridge for at least an hour, but preferably overnight.

Preheat the oven to 350°F. Line a rimmed baking sheet with parchment paper.

Place the marinated tofu on the baking sheet and bake for 25 to 30 minutes, flipping halfway through. Remove from the oven.

To make the roasted broccoli: Increase the oven temperature to 425°F. Line a baking sheet with parchment paper.

Toss the broccoli in the olive oil, garlic powder, and a sprinkle of salt and pepper. Arrange the broccoli on the baking sheet in an even layer. Roast for 15 to 20 minutes, until tender and starting to brown. Drizzle with fresh lemon juice. Serve the broccoli with the tofu.

VEGGIE CHEESE FRITTATA

Serves 3
Prep Time: 5 minutes
Cook Time: 18 minutes
Calories: 375 per serving
Carbs: 5g per serving

5 eggs
¼ cup whole or nondairy milk
½ teaspoon sea salt, plus more for the salad
¼ teaspoon black pepper, plus more for serving
¾ cup shredded cheddar cheese
¼ cup grated Parmesan cheese
½ cup cherry tomatoes, halved
½ cup diced bell pepper
3 cups fresh baby spinach, loosely packed
3 cups fresh arugula
Extra-virgin olive oil
3 tablespoons walnuts or other nut/seed
1 lemon

Preheat the oven to 400°F. Grease a medium baking dish (Pyrex or cast iron work well).

In a medium bowl, whisk the eggs, milk, salt, and pepper until smooth. Mix in the shredded cheddar, Parmesan, tomatoes, bell pepper, and spinach.

Pour the mixture into the baking dish and bake for 15 to 18 minutes, until the edges are set and the top is slightly browned.

Cut into four portions and serve over a bed of arugula dressed with a little olive oil, salt and pepper, 1 tablespoon walnuts, and fresh lemon juice.

BERRY YOGURT BARK

Serves 2
Prep Time: 5 minutes
Cook Time: 2 hours
Calories: 190 per serving
Carbs: 18g per serving

2 cups vanilla low-fat Greek yogurt
½ cup sliced fresh strawberries
½ cup fresh blueberries
2 teaspoons chia seeds

Line a rimmed baking sheet with parchment paper.

Pour the yogurt onto the baking sheet and spread it out evenly. Sprinkle with the strawberries, blueberries, and chia seeds.

Place in the freezer for 2 to 3 hours, or until firm. Break into chunks and enjoy!

WEEK 6 MEAL PLANS

MONDAY

Breakfast: Veggie Breakfast Skillet (page 205)

Lunch: Sriracha Cauliflower Chickpea Bake (page 208)

Dinner: Savory Crockpot Chili (page 207)

TUESDAY

Breakfast: Carrot Cake Breakfast Cookies (page 206)

Lunch: Sriracha Cauliflower Chickpea Bake (page 208)

Dinner: Black Bean Burger and Fries (page 209)

WEDNESDAY

Breakfast: Veggie Breakfast Skillet (page 205)

Lunch: Savory Crockpot Chili (page 207)

Dinner: Black Bean Burger and Fries (page 209)

THURSDAY

Breakfast: Carrot Cake Breakfast Cookies (page 206)

Lunch: Sriracha Cauliflower Chickpea Bake (page 208)

Dinner: Savory Crockpot Chili (page 207)

FRIDAY

Breakfast: Veggie Breakfast Skillet (page 205)

Lunch: Savory Crockpot Chili (page 207)

Dinner: Black Bean Burger and Fries (page 209)

SHOPPING LIST

PANTRY ITEMS

Olive oil spray
Extra-virgin olive oil
Avocado oil
Sriracha
Sea salt
Black pepper
Italian seasoning
Chili powder
Smoked paprika
Garlic powder

Baking powder
Ground cinnamon
Worcestershire sauce
⅓ cup sugar-free maple syrup
Apple cider vinegar
Honey
4 cups chicken bone broth
One 16-ounce jar Fresno chiles
Low-sodium soy sauce

PRODUCE

2 bananas
1 avocado
2 large sweet potatoes
2 yellow onions
2 red bell peppers
1 medium zucchini
1 cup spinach, loosely packed
1 head butter lettuce
1 large head cauliflower

½ cup cremini mushrooms
1 cup sliced baby bella mushrooms
2 medium carrots
½ cup frozen corn
2 Roma tomatoes
1 butternut squash
1 fresh jalapeño
1 head garlic
1 bunch fresh cilantro

PROTEINS

6 eggs
1 scoop of vanilla protein powder
1 pound ground chicken
¼ cup almond butter

⅓ cup plain low-fat Greek yogurt
One 15-ounce can chickpeas
One 15-ounce can black beans
1¾ cups cooked red lentils

OTHER

½ cup chopped pecans
1½ cups old-fashioned rolled oats
½ cup whole-wheat flour
½ cup oat flour

¼ cup ground flaxseed
⅓ cup mayonnaise
2 tablespoons raisins

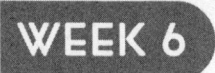

1. 2 tablespoons tahini and ½ cup sliced cucumber

2. ¾ cup Pumpkin Spice Roasted Chickpeas: Roast a can of chickpeas with 1 tablespoon of olive oil and some pumpkin pie spice seasoning

3. Ripe pear and ¼ cup whole-milk cottage cheese

4. 1 hard-boiled egg and ½ cup baby carrots

5. Hummus Avocado Toast (page 211)

VEGGIE BREAKFAST SKILLET

Serves 1
Prep Time: 10 minutes
Cook Time: 10 minutes
Calories: 306 per serving
Carbs: 16.5g per serving

Olive oil spray
½ cup frozen corn
¼ yellow onion, diced
½ red bell pepper, diced
1 cup baby spinach, loosely packed
½ cup cremini mushrooms, sliced
2 eggs
Sea salt and black pepper
¼ avocado, sliced
¼ jalapeño, seeded and thinly sliced

Spray a large nonstick skillet with olive oil spray and heat over medium heat. Place the corn, onion, red bell pepper, spinach, and mushrooms in the skillet and sauté until tender, about 5 minutes.

Crack the eggs into the skillet and sprinkle salt and pepper over the eggs and veggies. Cook until the whites are set and the yolks are slightly runny, 3 to 4 minutes.

Top with the avocado and jalapeño and serve warm.

CARROT CAKE BREAKFAST COOKIES

Makes 15 cookies; 3 cookies per serving
Prep Time: 20 minutes
Cook Time: 20 minutes
Calories: 365 per serving
Carbs: 37g per serving

Olive oil spray
½ cup whole-wheat flour
1 scoop vanilla protein powder
1½ cups old-fashioned rolled oats
¼ cup ground flaxseed
1 teaspoon baking powder
1 teaspoon ground cinnamon
½ teaspoon sea salt
2 medium carrots, grated
½ cup chopped pecans
2 tablespoons raisins
1 egg
2 bananas, mashed (can also substitute ½ cup unsweetened applesauce)
¼ cup almond butter
⅓ cup sugar-free maple syrup

Preheat the oven to 350°F. Grease a baking sheet with olive oil spray.

In a large mixing bowl, whisk together the flour, protein powder, oats, ground flaxseed, baking powder, cinnamon, and salt. Stir in the carrots, pecans, and raisins to combine.

In a separate medium bowl, combine the egg, bananas, almond butter, and sugar-free maple syrup. Whisk until blended. Pour the wet ingredients into the dry ingredients and mix until just combined.

Form 15 cookies out of the dough and place on the baking sheet.

Bake for 15 to 20 minutes, until the cookies are firm and golden. Let cool for 10 minutes, then enjoy!

Store leftover cookies in the fridge for up to 5 days. These also freeze well!

SAVORY CROCKPOT CHILI

Serves 4
Prep Time: 10 minutes
Cook Time: 5 hours
Calories: 325 per serving
Carbs: 21g per serving

1 tablespoon olive oil
3 cloves garlic, minced
1 pound ground chicken
2 cups peeled and chopped (½-inch cubes) butternut squash
2 Roma tomatoes, diced
1 medium zucchini, diced
1 cup sliced baby bella mushrooms
1 red bell pepper, diced
4 cups chicken bone broth
1 tablespoon Italian seasoning
½ teaspoon sea salt
¼ teaspoon black pepper

In a large skillet, heat the olive oil over medium heat. Add the garlic and cook for about 30 seconds.

Add the ground chicken and cook until no longer pink, 6 to 8 minutes. Transfer the chicken and garlic to the slow cooker.

Add the butternut squash, tomatoes, zucchini, mushrooms, and bell pepper to the slow cooker. Pour the bone broth over the chicken and vegetables and sprinkle the Italian seasoning, salt, and pepper on top.

Stir, cover, and cook on low for 5 hours, or until the vegetables are tender. Serve hot and enjoy!

SRIRACHA CAULIFLOWER CHICKPEA BAKE

Serves 3
Prep Time: 10 minutes
Cook Time: 35 minutes
Calories: 387 per serving
Carbs: 46 per serving

1 large head cauliflower, chopped into florets
1 yellow onion, chopped
One 15-ounce can chickpeas, drained, rinsed, and patted dry
¼ cup Fresno chiles, drained and patted dry
1 tablespoon avocado oil
½ teaspoon sea salt
¼ teaspoon ground black pepper
1½ cups cooked red lentils
3 tablespoons minced fresh cilantro

Creamy Sriracha Sauce

1 tablespoon sriracha
2 tablespoons low-sodium soy sauce
⅓ cup mayonnaise
⅓ cup plain low-fat Greek yogurt
1 tablespoon honey
2 teaspoons apple cider vinegar
2 garlic cloves, minced

Preheat the oven to 450°F. Line a baking pan with parchment paper.

Place the cauliflower, onion, chickpeas, and Fresno chiles on the prepared pan. Drizzle with the avocado oil and sprinkle with the salt and pepper. Stir to combine and bake for 20 to 25 minutes, until light golden brown. Allow to cool for 10 minutes, then pour into a large bowl.

Make the creamy sriracha sauce: In a small bowl, combine the sriracha, soy sauce, mayonnaise, Greek yogurt, honey, vinegar, and garlic.

Pour the sauce into the bowl with the cauliflower, onion, chickpeas, and chiles and toss to coat evenly. Serve each serving with ½ cup cooked red lentils, garnish with fresh minced cilantro, and enjoy warm.

BLACK BEAN BURGER AND FRIES

Serves 3
Prep Time: 15 minutes
Cook Time: 30 minutes
Calories: 406 per serving
Carbs: 51g per serving

Black Bean Burgers

One 15-ounce can black beans, rinsed, drained, and patted dry
½ cup oat flour
½ cup minced yellow onion
3 garlic cloves, minced
1 egg
1 tablespoon Worcestershire sauce
½ teaspoon garlic powder
1 teaspoon smoked paprika
1 teaspoon chili powder
¼ teaspoon sea salt
⅛ teaspoon ground black pepper
Avocado oil
1 head butter lettuce

Sweet Potato Fries

2 large sweet potatoes
2 tablespoons avocado oil
¼ teaspoon sea salt

To make the burgers: Place the black beans in a large bowl and mash them with a fork or potato masher until they are mostly mashed but there are still some larger pieces left. Mix in the oat flour, onion, and garlic.

In a medium bowl, whisk the egg, Worcestershire sauce, garlic powder, smoked paprika, chili powder, salt, and pepper until well combined.

Pour the egg mixture into the bowl with the black beans and stir until a dough-like consistency is formed.

(continued)

Divide the mixture into three equal patties.

Heat about 1 tablespoon avocado oil in a nonstick skillet over medium heat. Cook each patty for 5 to 8 minutes per side, until the burgers are browned and reach at least 160°F in the center.

Add desired toppings (such as no-sugar-added ketchup, sliced tomato, yellow mustard, or sliced red onion) and wrap each patty in butter lettuce leaves.

To make the fries: Preheat the oven to 425°F and line two large rimmed baking sheets with parchment paper.

Peel the sweet potatoes and cut them into fry-shaped pieces about ¼ inch wide and ¼ inch thick. Divide the fries between the two pans as evenly as possible, and try to space them out so they're not touching.

Drizzle with avocado oil, then sprinkle with the salt.

Bake for 30 minutes, flipping halfway through.

Serve the sweet potato fries with the burgers and enjoy.

HUMMUS AVOCADO TOAST

Serves 1
Prep Time: 1 minute
Cook Time: 3 minutes
Calories: 206 per serving
Carbs: 27g per serving

1 slice whole-grain bread, toasted
1 tablespoon hummus
3 thin cucumber slices
½ small radish, thinly sliced
¼ avocado, thinly sliced
1 small handful fresh arugula
¼ teaspoon fresh lemon juice
Red pepper flakes, to taste
Pinch of everything bagel seasoning

Spread the toast with hummus and top it with the cucumber, radish, and avocado. Top with the arugula, lemon juice, red pepper flakes, and everything bagel seasoning.

MEAL PLAN NOTES

IF YOU ARE NOT WORKING ON WEIGHT LOSS:

If you are not actively working on weight loss, choose two out of three of the following options:

→ Add one piece of fruit (or 1 cup chopped/sliced fruit) to any meal.

→ Double the portion size of your protein for any meal.

→ Add one extra snack per day from the snack list (this could also be a small low-carb dessert).

IF YOU ARE PREGNANT:

→ **In your first trimester:** No diet changes are required.

→ **In your second trimester:** Add one extra snack per day from the snack list (this could also be a small low-carb dessert).

→ **In your third trimester:** Add two extra snacks per day from the snack list (this could also be a small low-carb dessert).

Note: Sometimes our appetites and eating patterns get crazy during pregnancy! Absolutely no worries if you need to add more snacks or to change the portion sizes of your protein/veggies/fats/carbs to be bigger or smaller! Do the best you can and listen to your body, mama!

IF YOU ARE BREASTFEEDING:

→ If you're exclusively breastfeeding, follow the guidelines above for the third trimester.

→ If you are half breastfeeding and half formula feeding, follow the guidelines above for the second trimester.

ACKNOWLEDGMENTS

I would like to thank my virtual assistant-turned-chief-of-staff, but also right-hand woman, Mara Davey, for her continuous support and dedication to my practice, this book, and all women with PCOS. You are truly an angel, and I wish I could clone you twice.

Thank you to my brilliant team of editors at Rodale. You all had to suffer through endless recipe retesting and revisions, and I am so thankful.

I would also like to thank my writing coach Isabella Massucci; you really brought this book to life, helped me pull out the right stories, and gave me the courage, organization, and structure to take the leap and actually follow through with it.

Thank you to Amanda Bernardi; I am so glad we got the opportunity to work together on this beast of a book!

Special thanks to my dishwasher for speeding up the scrubbing of the mountain of dirty dishes I accumulated; you're the real MVP.

REFERENCES

Agarwal, Sanjay K., Charles Chapron, Linda C. Giudice, Marc R. Laufer, Nicholas Leyland, Stacey A. Missmer, Sukhbir S. Singh, and Hugh S. Taylor. "Clinical Diagnosis of Endometriosis: A Call to Action." *American Journal of Obstetrics and Gynecology* 220, no. 4 (April 2019): 354. e1–12. https://doi.org/10.1016/j.ajog.2018.12.039.

Aghasi, Mohadeseh, Mahdieh Golzarand, Sakineh Shab-Bidar, Azadeh Aminianfar, Mahsa Omidian, and Fatemeh Taheri. "Dairy Intake and Acne Development: A Meta-Analysis of Observational Studies." *Clinical Nutrition* 38, no. 3 (May 8, 2018): 1067–75. https://doi.org/10.1016/j.clnu.2018.04.015.

Amini, Leila. "Antioxidants and Management of Polycystic Ovary Syndrome in Iran: A Systematic Review of Clinical Trials." PubMed Central (PMC), January 1, 2015. https://www.ncbi.nlm.nih.gov/pmc/articles/PMC4306978/.

"Anatomy of the Endocrine System." Johns Hopkins Medicine. November 19, 2019. https://www.hopkinsmedicine.org/health/wellness-and-prevention/anatomy-of-the-endocrine-system.

Bajekal, Nitu, and Rohini Bajekal. *Living PCOS Free: How to Regain Your Hormonal Health with Polycystic Ovarian Syndrome.* London: Hammersmith Books Limited, 2022.

Baskin, Laurence S., Joel Shen, Adriane Sinclair, Mei Cao, Xin Liu, Ge Liu, Dylan Isaacson, Maya Overland, Yang Li, and Gerald R. Cunha. "Development of the Human Penis and Clitoris." *Differentiation* 103 (September 1, 2018): 74–85. https://doi.org/10.1016/j.diff.2018.08.001.

Borenstein, Jeff E., Bonnie B. Dean, Jean Endicott, John Wong, Candace Brown, Vivian Dickerson, and Kimberly A. Yonkers. "Health and Economic Impact of the Premenstrual Syndrome." *Journal of Reproductive Medicine* 48 (July 2023): 515–24. https://pubmed.ncbi.nlm.nih.gov/12953326/.

Canivenc-Lavier, Marie-Chantal, and Catherine Bennetau-Pelissero. "Phytoestrogens and Health Effects." *Nutrients* 15, no. 2 (January 9, 2023): 317. https://doi.org/10.3390/nu15020317.

Cappelletti, Simone, Daria Piacentino, Gabriele Sani, and Mariarosaria Aromatario. "Caffeine: Cognitive and Physical Performance Enhancer or Psychoactive Drug?" *Current Neuropharmacology* 13, no. 1 (January 2015): 71–88. https://doi.org/10.2174/1570159X13666141210215655.

Cardinale, Vincenzo, Elisa Lepore, Sabrina Basciani, Salvatore Artale, Mauritzio Nordio, Mariano Bizzarri, and Vittorio Unfer. "Positive Effects of α-Lactalbumin in the Management of Symptoms of Polycystic Ovary Syndrome." *Nutrients* 14, no. 15 (August 6, 2022): 3220. https://doi.org/10.3390/nu14153220.

Cosmacini, G. "Long Art: The History of Medicine from Antiquity to the Present." Rome: Oxford University Press, 1997.

Dusenbery, Maya. "Everybody Was Telling Me There Was Nothing Wrong." *Health Gap,* 2019. https://www.bbc.com/future/article/20180523-how-gender-bias-affects-your-healthcare.

El-Hamamsy, Dina, Chanel Parmar, Stephanie Shoop-Worrall, and Fiona M. Reid. "Public Understanding of Female Genital Anatomy and Pelvic Organ Prolapse (POP); a Questionnaire-Based Pilot Study." *International Urogynecology Journal* 33, no. 2 (March 31, 2021): 309–18. https://doi.org/10.1007/s00192-021-04727-9.

Esposito, Katherine, and Dario Giugliano. "Diet and Inflammation: A Link to Metabolic and Cardiovascular Diseases." *European Heart Journal* 27, no. 1 (January 2006): 15–20. https://doi.org/10.1093/eurheartj/ehi605.

Food and Nutrition Service, USDA. "Nutrition Standards in the National School Lunch and School Breakfast Programs." *Govinfo.Gov.* Department of Agriculture, January 13, 2011.

Fourquet, Jessica, Ninet Sinaii, Pamela Stratton, Fareed Khayel, Carolina Alvarez-Garriga, Manuel Bayona, Mary Lou Ballweg, and Idhaliz Flores. "Characteristics of Women with Endometriosis from the USA and Puerto Rico." *Journal of Endometriosis and Pelvic Pain Disorders* 7, no. 4 (October–December 2015): 129–35. https://doi.org/10.5301/je.5000224.

Gibson, Claire L. "Hormones and Behaviour: A Psychological Approach." *Perspectives in Biology and Medicine,* 53, 152–55 (2010).

González, Fidelina. "Inflammation in Polycystic Ovary Syndrome: Underpinning of Insulin Resistance and Ovarian Dysfunction." *Steroids* 77, no. 4 (March 10, 2012): 300–05. https://doi.org/10.1016/j.steroids.2011.12.003.

Grant, Paul. "Spearmint Herbal Tea Has Significant Anti-Androgen Effects in Polycystic Ovarian Syndrome. A Randomized Controlled Trial." *Phytotherapy Research* 24, no. 2 (July 7, 2009): 186–88. https://doi.org/10.1002/ptr.2900.

Greenwood, Eleni A., Lauri A. Pasch, Marcelle I. Cedars, Richard S. Legro, Esther Eisenberg, Heather G. Huddleston, and Eunice Kennedy Shriver National Institute of Child Health and Human Development Reproductive Medicine Network. "Insulin Resistance Is Associated with Depression Risk in Polycystic Ovary Syndrome." *Fertility and Sterility* 110, no. 1 (July 1, 2018): 27–34. https://doi.org/10.1016/j.fertnstert.2018.03.009.

Gudipally, Pratyusha R., and Gyanendra K. Sharma. "Premenstrual Syndrome." PubMed. Treasure Island (FL): StatPearls Publishing. 2021. https://www.ncbi.nlm.nih.gov/books/NBK560698/.

Hamid, Amr Mohamed Salah El Din Abdel, Wael A. Ismail Madkour, and Tamer Farouk Borg. "Inositol versus Metformin Administration in Polycystic Ovary Syndrome Patients." *Evidence Based Women's Health Journal* 5, no. 2 (May 2015): 61–66. https://doi.org/10.1097/01.ebx.0000466599.33293.cf.

Han, Quixin, Juan Wang, Weiping Li, Zi-Jiang Chen, and Yanzhi Du. "Androgen-Induced Gut Dysbiosis Disrupts Glucolipid Metabolism and Endocrinal Functions in Polycystic Ovary Syndrome." *Microbiome* 9, no. 1 (May 6, 2021): 101. https://doi.org/10.1186/s40168-021-01046-5.

Herrera, Alexandra Ycaza, Shawn E. Nielsen, and Mara Mather. "Stress-Induced Increases in Progesterone and Cortisol in Naturally Cycling Women." *Neurobiology of Stress* 3 (June 1, 2016): 96–104. https://doi.org/10.1016/j.ynstr.2016.02.006.

Hodskinson, Michael R., Alice Bolner, Koichi Sato, Ashley N. Kamimae-Lanning, Koos Rooijers, Merlijn Witte, Mohan Mahesh, Jan Silhan, Maya Petek, David M. Williams, Jop Kind, Jason W. Chin, Ketan J. Patel, and Puck Knipscheer. "Alcohol-Derived DNA Crosslinks Are Repaired by Two Distinct Mechanisms." *Nature* 579, no. 7800 (March 2020): 603–08. https://doi.org/10.1038/s41586-020-2059-5.

Holick, Michael F., Neil C. Binkley, Heike A. Bischoff-Ferrari, Catherine M. Gordon, David A. Hanley, Robert P. Heaney, M. Hassan Murad, Connie M. Weaver; Endocrine Society. "Evaluation, Treatment, and Prevention of Vitamin D Deficiency: An Endocrine Society Clinical Practice Guideline." *Journal of Clinical Endocrinology & Metabolism* 96, no. 7 (July 2011): 1911–30. https://doi.org/10.1210/jc.2011-0385.

Hong, Xiang, Pengfei Qin, Jiechen Yin, Yong Shi, Yan Xuan, Zhengqi Chen, Xu Zhou, Hong Yu, Danhong Peng, and Bei Wang. "Clinical Manifestations of Polycystic Ovary Syndrome and Associations with the Vaginal Microbiome: A Cross-Sectional Based Exploratory Study." *Frontiers in Endocrinology* 12 (April 23, 2021): 662725. https://doi.org/10.3389/fendo.2021.662725.

Johnson, Sarah, Lorrae Marriott, and Michael J. Zinaman. "Can Apps and Calendar Methods Predict Ovulation with Accuracy?" *Current Medical Research and Opinion* 34, no. 9 (May 25, 2018): 1587–94. https://doi.org/10.1080/03007995.2018.1475348.

Juanola-Falgarona, Martí, Jordi Salas-Salvadó, Núria Ibarrola-Jurado, Antoni Rabassa-Soler, Andrés Díaz-López, Marta Guasch-Ferré, Pablo Hernández-Alonso, Rafael Balanza, and Mònica Bulló. "Effect of the Glycemic Index of the Diet on Weight Loss, Modulation of Satiety, Inflammation, and Other Metabolic Risk Factors: A Randomized Controlled Trial." *American Journal of Clinical Nutrition* 100, no. 1 (July 2014): 27–35. https://doi.org/10.3945/ajcn.113.081216.

Khan, Muhammad Jaseem, Anwar Ullah, and Sulman Basit. "Genetic Basis of Polycystic Ovary Syndrome (PCOS): Current Perspectives." *Application of Clinical Genetics,* 12 (December 24, 2019): 249–60. https://doi.org/10.2147/TACG.S200341.

Knudtson, Jennifer. "Menstrual Cycle." Merck Manuals Consumer Version. Merck Manuals. 2018. https://www.merckmanuals.com/home/women-s-health-issues/biology-of-the-female-reproductive-system/menstrual-cycle.

Kuchenbecker, Shari Young, Sarah D. Pressman, Jared Celniker, Karen M. Grewen, Kenneth D. Sumida, Naveen Jonathan, Brendan Everett, and George M. Slavich. "Oxytocin, Cortisol, and Cognitive Control During Acute and Naturalistic Stress." *Stress* 24, no. 4 (July 2021): 370–83.

Lagowska, Karolina. "The Relationship Between Vitamin D Status and the Menstrual Cycle in Young Women: A Preliminary Study." *Nutrients* 10, no. 11 (November 11, 2018): 1729. https://www.ncbi.nlm.nih.gov/pmc/articles/PMC6265788/.

Lee, Iris, Laura G. Cooney, Shailly Saini, Mary D. Sammel, Kelly C. Allison, and Anuja Dokras. "Increased Odds of Disordered Eating in Polycystic Ovary Syndrome: A Systematic Review and Meta-Analysis." *Eating and Weight Disorders* 24, no. 5 (October 2019): 787–97. https://doi.org/10.1007/s40519-018-0533-y.

Lee, J., V. Taneja, and R. Vassallo. "Cigarette Smoking and Inflammation: Cellular and Molecular Mechanisms." *Journal of Dental Research* 91, no. 2 (August 29, 2011): 142–49. https://doi.org/10.1177/0022034511421200.

Liao, Wan-Ting, Jing-Yang Huang, Ming-Tsung Lee, Yu-Cih Yang, and Chun-Chi Wu. "Higher Risk of Type 2 Diabetes in Young Women with Polycystic Ovary Syndrome: A 10-Year Retrospective Cohort Study." *World Journal of Diabetes* 13, no. 3 (March 15, 2022): 240–50. https://doi.org/10.4239/wjd.v13.i3.240.

Lizneva, Daria, Larisa Suturina, Walidah Walker, Soumia Brakta, Larisa Gavrilova-Jordan, and Ricardo Azziz. "Criteria, Prevalence, and Phenotypes of Polycystic Ovary Syndrome." *Fertility and Sterility* 106, no. 1 (July 2016): 6–15. https://doi.org/10.1016/j.fertnstert.2016.05.003.

Lovallo, William R., Noha H. Farag, Andrea S. Vincent, Terrie L. Thomas, and Michael F. Wilson. "Cortisol Responses to Mental Stress, Exercise, and Meals Following Caffeine Intake in Men and Women." *Pharmacology,*

Biochemistry and Behavior 83, no. 3 (March 2006): 441–47. https://doi.org/10.1016/j.pbb.2006.03.005.

Lu, Kuan-Ta, Yu-Cheng Ho, Chen-Lin Chang, Kuo-Chung Lan, Cheng-Chun Wu, and Yu-Ting Su. "Evaluation of Bodily Pain Associated with Polycystic Ovary Syndrome: A Review of Health-Related Quality of Life and Potential Risk Factors." *Biomedicines* 10, no. 12 (December 9, 2022): 3197. https://doi.org/10.3390/biomedicines10123197.

Masaki, Hitoshi. "Role of Antioxidants in the Skin: Anti-Aging Effects." *Journal of Dermatological Science* 58, no. 2 (July 10, 2010): 85–90. https://doi.org/10.1016/j.jdermsci.2010.03.003.

Mayo Clinic Staff. "Low-Carb Diet: Can It Help You Lose Weight?" Mayo Clinic, November 15, 2022, https://www.mayoclinic.org/healthy-lifestyle/weight-loss/in-depth/low-carb-diet/art-20045831.

Meixiong, James, Cristina Ricco, Chirag Vasavda, and Byron K. Ho. "Diet and Acne: A Systematic Review." *Journal of the American Academy of Dermatology International* 7 (March 29, 2022): 95–112. https://doi.org/10.1016/j.jdin.2022.02.012.

Mikulic, Matej. "Review of Number of Metformin Prescriptions in the U.S. from 2004 to 2021." *Statistica* (November 1, 2024). https://www.statista.com/statistics/780332/metformin-hydrochloride-prescriptions-number-in-the-us/.

Mumford, Sunni L., Jorge E. Chavarro, Cuilin Zhang, Neil J. Perkins, Lindsey A. Sjaarda, Anna Z. Pollack, Karen C. Schliep, Kara A. Michels, Shvetha M. Zarek, Torie C. Plowden, Rose G. Radin, Lynne C. Messer, Robyn A. Frankel, and Jean Wactawski-Wende. "Dietary Fat Intake and Reproductive Hormone Concentrations and Ovulation in Regularly Menstruating Women." *American Journal of Clinical Nutrition* 103, no. 3 (March 2016): 868–77. doi: 10.3945/ajcn.115.119321.

Nagoski, Emily. *Come as You Are: The Surprising New Science That Will Transform Your Sex Life.* New York: Simon and Schuster, 2022.

Nagoski, Emily, and Amelia Nagoski. *Burnout: The Secret to Solving the Stress Cycle.* New York: Random House, 2019.

Nnoaham, Kelechi E., Lone Hummelshoj, Premila Webster, Thomas d'Hooghe, Fiorenzo de Cicco Nardone, Carlo de Cicco Nardone, Crispin Jenkinson, Stephen H. Kennedy, and Krina T. Zondervan; World Endometriosis Research Foundation Global Study of Women's Health Consortium. "Impact of Endometriosis on Quality of Life and Work Productivity: A Multicenter Study Across Ten Countries." *Fertility and Sterility* 96, no. 2 (August 2011): 366–73.

Nutrition Source, The. "Antioxidants." March 3, 2021. https://www.hsph.harvard.edu/nutritionsource/antioxidants/.

Office on Women's Health. "Polycystic Ovary Syndrome." Womenshealth.gov. February 22, 2021. https://www.womenshealth.gov/a-z-topics/polycystic-ovary-syndrome.

Pahwa, Roma. "Chronic Inflammation." StatPearls—NCBI Bookshelf. August 7, 2023. https://www.ncbi.nlm.nih.gov/books/NBK493173/.

Palmery, M., A. Saraceno, A. Vaiarelli, and G. Carlomagno. "Oral Contraceptives and Changes in Nutritional Requirements." *European Review for Medical and Pharmacological Sciences* 17, no. 13 (July 2013): 1804–13. https://pubmed.ncbi.nlm.nih.gov/23852908/.

"PCOS (Polycystic Ovary Syndrome) and Diabetes." Centers for Disease Control and Prevention. August 12, 2022. https://www.cdc.gov/diabetes/basics/pcos.html.

Petersen, Max C., and Gerald I. Shulman. "Mechanisms of Insulin Action and Insulin Resistance." *Physiological Reviews* 98, no. 4 (October 1, 2018): 2133–223. https://doi.org/10.1152/physrev.00063.2017.

Petersen, Nicole, Alexandra Touroutoglou, Joseph M. Andreano, and Larry Cahill. "Oral Contraceptive Pill Use Is Associated with Localized Decreases in Cortical Thickness." *Human Brain Mapping* 36, no. 7 (July 2015): 2644–54. https://doi.org/10.1002/hbm.22797.

Professional, Cleveland Clinic Medical. "Visceral Fat." Cleveland Clinic, n.d. https://my.clevelandclinic.org/health/diseases/24147-visceral-fat.

Rapkin, Andrea J., and Sharon A. Winer. "Premenstrual Syndrome and Premenstrual Dysphoric Disorder: Quality of Life and Burden of Illness." *Expert Review of Pharmacoeconomics & Outcomes Research* 9, no. 2 (April 2009): 157–70. https://doi.org/10.1586/erp.09.14.

Rehm, Jürgen, Kevin D. Shield, and Elisabete Weiderpass. "Alcohol Consumption. A Leading Risk Factor for Cancer." *Chemico-Biological Interactions* 331 (November 1, 2020): 109280. https://doi.org/10.1016/j.cbi.2020.109280.

Rodsky, Eve. *Fair Play: A Game-Changing Solution for When You Have Too Much Do (and More Life to Live).* New York: G.P. Putnam's Sons, 2019.

Royal College of Obstetricians and Gynaecologists. "Long-Term Consequences of Polycystic Ovary Syndrome." *Green-top Guideline No. 33*, November 2014. www.rcog.org.uk/globalassets/documents/guidelines/gtg_33.pdf.

Rubin, Eugene H., and Charles F. Zorumski. *Adult Psychiatry.* Malden, MA: Blackwell Publishing, 2005.

Rudnicka, Ewa, Katarzyna Suchta, Monika Grymowicz, Anna Calik-Ksepka, Katarzyna Smolarczyk, A. M. Duszewska, Roman Smolarczyk, and Błażej Męczekalski. "Chronic Low Grade Inflammation in Pathogenesis of PCOS." *International Journal of Molecular Sciences* 22, no. 7 (April 6, 2021): 3789. https://doi.org/10.3390/ijms22073789.

Ruegsegger, Gregory N., and Frank W. Booth. "Health Benefits of Exercise." *Cold Spring Harbor Perspectives in Medicine* (July 2018): a029694. doi:10.1101/cshperspect

.a029694. https://www.ncbi.nlm.nih.gov/pmc/articles/PMC6027933/.

Sadehi, Hosna Mohammad, Ida Adeli, Daniela Calina, Anca Oana Docea, Taraneh Mousavi, Marzieh Daniali, Shekoufeh Nikfar, Aristidis Tsatsakis, and Mohammad Abdollahi. "Polycystic Ovary Syndrome: A Comprehensive Review of Pathogenesis, Management, and Drug Repurposing." *International Journal of Molecular Sciences* 23, no. 2 (January 6, 2022): 583. https://doi.org/10.3390/ijms23020583.

Sam, Susan. "Obesity and Polycystic Ovary Syndrome." *Obesity Management* 3, no. 2 (April 2007): 69–73. https://doi.org/10.1089/obe.2007.0019.

Samulowitz, Anke, Ida Gremyr, Erik Eriksson, and Gunnel Hensing. "'Brave Men' and 'Emotional Women': A Theory-Guided Literature Review on Gender Bias in Health Care and Gendered Norms Towards Patients with Chronic Pain." *Pain Research & Management* (February 25, 2018): 6358624. https://doi.org/10.1155/2018/6358624.

Sapolsky, Robert M. *Why Zebras Don't Get Ulcers*. New York: W. H. Freeman & Co., 1994. http://ci.nii.ac.jp/ncid/BB08461890.

Sears, Barry. "Anti-Inflammatory Diets for Obesity and Diabetes." *Journal of the American College of Nutrition* 28 (August 2009): 482S–91S. https://doi.org/10.1080/07315724.2009.10718115.

Shahdadian, Farnaz, Reza Ghiasvand, Behnood Abbasi, Awat Feizi, Parvane Saneei, and Zahra Shahshahan. "Association Between Major Dietary Patterns and Polycystic Ovary Syndrome: Evidence from a Case-Control Study." *Applied Physiology, Nutrition, and Metabolism = Physiologie Appliquee, Nutrition et Metabolisme* 44, no. 1 (January 2019): 52–58. https://doi.org/10.1139/apnm-2018-0145.

Sharma, Ashish, Vishal Madaan, and Frederick D. Petty. "Exercise for Mental Health." *Primary Care Companion to the Journal of Clinical Psychiatry* 8, no. 2 (2006): 106.

Sidra, Syeda, Muhammad Haseeb Tariq, Muhammad Junaid Farrukh, and Muhammad Mohsin. "Evaluation of Clinical Manifestations, Health Risks, and Quality of Life Among Women with Polycystic Ovary Syndrome." *PLoS One* 14, no. 10 (October 11, 2019): e0223329. https://doi.org/10.1371/journal.pone.0223329.

Stener-Victorin, Elisabet, Vasantha Padmanabhan, Kristy A. Walters, Rebecca E. Campbell, Anna Benrick, Paolo Giacobini, Daniel A. Dumesic, and David H. Abbott. "Animal Models to Understand the Etiology and Pathophysiology of Polycystic Ovary Syndrome." *Endocrine Reviews* 41, no. 4 (July 1, 2020): bnaa010.

Tafet, G. E., M. Toister-Achituv, and M. Shinitzky. "Enhancement of Serotonin Uptake by Cortisol: A Possible Link Between Stress and Depression." *Cognitive, Affective, & Behavioral Neuroscience* 1, no. 1 (March, 2001): 96–104. https://doi.org/10.3758/cabn.1.1.96.

Tasca, Cecilia, Mariangela Rapetti, Mauro Giovanni Carta, and Bianca Fadda. "Women and Hysteria in the History of Mental Health." *Clinical Practice and Epidemiology in Mental Health* 8 (October 19, 2012): 110–19. https://doi.org/10.2174/1745017901208010110.

Teede, Helena J., Marie L. Misso, Michael F. Costello, Anuja Dokras, Joop Laven, Lisa Moran, Terhi Piltonen, and Robert J. Norman, on behalf of the International PCOS Network. "Recommendations from the International Evidence-Based Guideline for the Assessment and Management of Polycystic Ovary Syndrome." *Human Reproduction* 33, no. 9 (2018): 1602–18.

Thomson, Rebecca L., Simon Spedding, and Jonathan D. Buckley. "Vitamin D in the Aetiology and Management of Polycystic Ovary Syndrome." *Clinical Endocrinology* 77, no. 3 (August 14, 2012): 343–50. https://doi.org/10.1111/j.1365-2265.2012.04434.x.

Titus-Lay, Erika, Tony Joseph Eid, Tiffany-Jade Kreys, Bo Xuan Joshua Chu, and Ashim Malhotra. "Trichotillomania Associated with 25-hydroxy Vitamin D Deficiency: A Case Report." *Mental Health Clinician* 10, no. 1 (January 9, 2020): 38–43.

U.S. Department of Agriculture and U.S. Department of Health and Human Services. Dietary Guidelines for Americans, 2020–25. 9th ed. Washington, D.C.: December 2020.

Wang, H. Joe, Samir Zakhari, and M. Katherine Jung. "Alcohol, Inflammation, and Gut-Liver-Brain Interactions in Tissue Damage and Disease Development." *World Journal of Gastroenterology* 16, no. 11 (March 21, 2010): 1304–13. https://doi.org/10.3748/wjg.v16.i11.1304.

Xing, Liwei, Jinlong Xu, Yuanyuan Wei, Yang Chen, Haina Zhuang, Wei Tang, Shun Yu, Junbao Zhang, Guochen Yin, Ruirui Wang, Rong Zhao, and Dongdong Qin. "Depression in Polycystic Ovary Syndrome: Focusing on Pathogenesis and Treatment." *Frontiers in Psychiatry* 13 (August 21, 2022): 1001484. https://doi.org/10.3389/fpsyt.2022.1001484.

Yuan, Xiaojie, Jiping Wang, Shuo Yang, Mei Gao, Lingxia Cao, Xumei Li, Dongxu Hong, Suyan Tian, and Chenglin Sun. "Effect of the Ketogenic Diet on Glycemic Control, Insulin Resistance, and Lipid Metabolism in Patients with T2DM: A Systematic Review and Meta-Analysis." *Nutrition & Diabetes* 10, no. 1 (November 30, 2020): 38. https://doi.org/10.1038/s41387-020-00142-z.

Zehravi, Mehrukh, Mudasir Maqbool, and Irfat Ara. "Depression and Anxiety in Women with Polycystic Ovarian Syndrome: A Literature Survey." *International Journal of Adolescent Medicine and Health* 33, no. 6 (August 2021). https://doi.org/10.1515/ijamh-2021-0092.

INDEX

ovulation
  benefits of, 30
  cycle, 55–56, 58
  irregular/absent, 14, 29–30
  myths about, 63–64
  progesterone production, 53, 55–56, 58
  reasons for irregular, 30
  regulating, 9
  stress and, 72
oxytocin, 94
Ozempic, 86

pain
  chronic, 27
  myths about, 45
  normalization of, 28
parabens, 81
parasympathetic nervous system, 70
patient rights, 42–43
patriarchy, 25, 27, 78
PCOS. *See* polycystic ovary syndrome
PCOS Boss Academy, 6
PCOS plate method, 135–137
Peanut Tofu Bowl, 198–199
pepperoni
  Zucchini Pizza Bites, 189
periods
  case study, 47–49
  cycle, 55–60
  hormones, 53–55
  irregular/absent, 24, 29
  myths about, 63–64
  ovulation and, 56
  PMS, 60
  stress and, 71–72
  tracking, 102
Pesto Sheet Pan Chicken and Veggies, 181
PFF (Protein! Fat! Fiber!) diet, 87, 93
phosphorus, 126
phthalates, 81
phytic acid, 128
phytoestrogens, 79
the Pill, 9, 43–44, 60–63, 77–78
Pita, Greek, 188

Pizza Bites, Zucchini, 189
plastics, 81
Plato, 26
PMS, 60, 63
polycystic ovary syndrome (PCOS)
  about, 20
  causes of, 23–24
  diagnosis, 8, 14–15, 23, 43–45
  health risks, 5, 7
  lab tests, 40–41
  myths about, 44–45
  prevalence of, 4, 20
  symptoms, 7, 8, 18, 24–25, 29–39, 83, 96–97
polyphenols, 129
pork
  Egg Roll in a Bowl, 160
  Garlic Butter Pork Skillet, 180
Portobello Baked Eggs, 175
potassium, 124
potatoes
  Pesto Sheet Pan Chicken and Veggies, 181
  Sheet Pan Chicken, 197
prediabetes, 16, 17
pregnancy
  difficulty getting pregnant, 19, 33–34
  health and, 44
  meal plan and, 212
  myths about, 63–64
  ovulation and, 55–56
probiotics, 96, 98
progesterone, 52, 53, 55–56, 58–59, 80
prolactin, 41
proteins, 33, 112, 115–116, 130, 136
Pumpkin Pie Yogurt, 195

quercetin, 97
quinoa
  One-Pan Southwest Shrimp and Asparagus, 159

rice
  Egg Roll in a Bowl, 160
  Mediterranean Baked Salmon, 170–171

· · · · · **ABOUT THE AUTHOR** · · · · ·

CORY RUTH is a registered dietitian nutritionist and women's health expert. Cory is the founder and principal of The Women's Dietitian and Instagram account, @thewomensdietitian, a private practice and digital platform for women seeking nutrition support for hormone balance, PCOS, fertility, and weight management. She specializes in PCOS and nutrition therapy for infertility and assisted reproductive technology.